MW00458629

TINY
PEP
TALKS

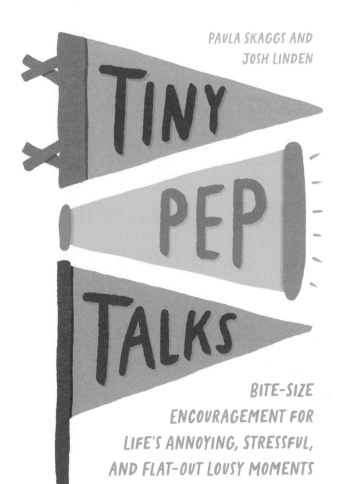

PAULA SKAGGS AND
JOSH LINDEN

TINY

PEP

TALKS

BITE-SIZE
ENCOURAGEMENT FOR
LIFE'S ANNOYING, STRESSFUL,
AND FLAT-OUT LOUSY MOMENTS

QUIRK BOOKS
PHILADELPHIA

Library of Congress Cataloging-in-Publication Data
Names: Skaggs, Paula, author. | Linden, Josh, author.
Title: Tiny pep talks : bite-size encouragement for life's annoying, stressful, and flat-out lousy moments / Paula Skaggs and Josh Linden.
Description: Philadelphia, PA : Quirk Books, [2024] | Summary: "A collection of humorous pep talks to encourage readers to face everyday challenges, in forms ranging from words of advice and fill-in-the-blank letters to songs and crosswords"—Provided by publisher.
Identifiers: LCCN 2024018100 (print) | LCCN 2024018101 (ebook) | ISBN 9781683694441 (hardcover) | ISBN 9781683694458 (ebook)
Subjects: LCSH: Encouragement. | Life skills. Classification: LCC BF637.E53 S47 2024 (print) | LCC BF637.E53 (ebook) | DDC 155.4/192—dc23/eng/20240502
LC record available at https://lccn.loc.gov/2024018100
LC ebook record available at https://lccn.loc.gov/2024018101

ISBN: 978-1-68369-444-1

Printed in China

Typeset in California Oranges and Quiet Sans

Designed by Andie Reid
Production management by Mandy Sampson

Quirk Books
215 Church Street
Philadelphia, PA 19106
quirkbooks.com

10 9 8 7 6 5 4 3 2 1

FSC
www.fsc.org
MIX
Paper | Supporting
responsible forestry
FSC® C008047

For Nora, David, and our parents,
and all their love, support,
and pep talks (both big and small)
along the way

FOR WHEN YOU'RE ABOUT TO READ A BOOK

A little birdie told us that you're about to read a book.

(It was the employee at the bookstore you just got this from and, frankly, we were surprised that they called us, too!)

Maybe the book in question is a special "Double the Length" edition of *Infinite Jest*. Or maybe, just maybe, it's a little book of encouraging pep talks for some of life's predicaments.

Whatever the book, remember that reading—a very noble pastime—is a marathon, not a sprint. Stay hydrated. Pack snacks. Treat yourself to a few minutes on your phone every so often, just to see if that one person from high school is up to anything new. The Pizza Hut Book It! reading program is (probably) not giving you a personal pan pizza for finishing, so there's no reason to rush. (But, you know, treat yourself to one anyway. You deserve it!)

LeVar Burton would be proud—and we are, too.

You're gonna do great.

CONTENTS

YOU IN THE WORLD

YOU & WORK

YOU & ROMANCE

YOU & THE BIG STUFF

An Introduction to TINY PEP TALKS

FREQUENTLY ASKED QUESTIONS

> ### HEY, SO WHAT IS THIS THING?

What a great question. You're absolutely crushing it right out of the gate!

This is *Tiny Pep Talks: Bite-Size Encouragement for Life's Annoying, Stressful, and Flat-Out Lousy Moments.* (It's also a book, although we suspect that you've figured that part out already.)

Here's the deal: It's easy to find someone to give you a pep talk for life's biggest moments. Folks line up to tell you "You've got this!" before the big job interview or as you head out onto the field to make the game-winning kick at the Super Bowl. (You know, universal experiences.)

And then there's the other 99.999 percent of the time.

We've all needed a little extra push to get through mundane, everyday obstacles—like when you're about to leave the house for a party where you don't know anyone (page 68) or when you have to get that boring work thing done (page 110).

That's where we come in. Within these pages, you'll find eighty-plus brief (or brief-ish) pep talks to get you through those everyday frustrations.

You can do the hard things—there's a thousand self-help books for that. But this book is here to remind you that you can also do the regular things, the annoying things, and the small things that somehow feel immensely overwhelming.

HOW EXACTLY DO I USE THIS BOOK?

Another great question. They should hire you to interview celebrities on *20/20*!

There are really no wrong answers here. Read the whole thing at once for an extra big dose of pep talks, storing them up in your brain for whenever you need them! Have a tailor alter your jeans so this book fits perfectly in your back pockets, so you can pull it out whenever awkward situations arise! Or memorize the whole book so you can recite it to your loved ones word for word whenever they need it! The world is your oyster!

(We also think it makes a great gift, a terrific coaster, and a fairly decent boomerang, as long as you don't care about it coming back to you.)

WHO THE HECK ARE YOU TO TELL ME WHAT TO DO?

Wow, not afraid to question authority—admirable!

We're Paula and Josh, the writers of this book (that's why they let us put our names on the cover). We're also comedians, card game creators, pretty big Bruce Springsteen fans, and two people who have been through hundreds (if not thousands) of totally normal yet somehow also wildly stressful situations, just like you.

We don't have PhDs in advanced humanistic psychology. We've never hosted a glitzy self-improvement TV show. We can't even send a text without overthinking every single word. But what we do have is an earnest outlook on life, and a firm belief that you are absolutely capable of conquering that annoying thing you have to do today.

Think of us as your constant pocket cheerleader, only with fewer pom-poms and even more exclamation marks!!!! We're the friends who will never judge you for rehearsing small talk in your head before a phone call or scream-crying as you parallel park—because we've been there, too.

> ### OKAY, FINE—I GUESS I COULD USE A PEP TALK OR TWO. WHAT'S NEXT?

Pragmatic *and* proactive. You're going places, kid!

Turn the page. Then turn the one after that, and the one after that, and the one after that. Keep turning until you're ready to conquer the world—or at least until you're ready to conquer that daunting work email.

You've got this.

YOU
AT
HOME

Being home is GREAT. That place has everything: Your favorite spatula! Your bed! Your second-favorite spatula! But it's also filled with a slew of potential pitfalls. Whatever you encounter, we've got you covered.

FOR WHEN IT'S TIME TO GET OFF THE COUCH AND GO TO BED

Okay, buster—the jig is up.

It's past your bedtime, yet here you are: on the couch, barely awake, with no intention of getting up and going to bed.

This is a classic case of Newton's first law of motion: objects at rest stay on the couch. We have a suspicion that you're scrolling on your phone while somehow also mindlessly watching a show you've already lost interest in, simply because the gravitational pull of the couch is too strong. So you need to make getting up and into bed as easy as possible.

Here's what you're going to do (and what we're confident you *can* do): get up and go to bed.

And here's what you're not going to do (and what we're confident you *wouldn't* have done anyway): anything else beyond that.

Too tired to wash your face? We'll worry about it tomorrow! Don't want to brush your teeth? Molars aren't that useful anyway! Too sleepy to put on PJs? Your jeans are plenty comfy!

The one and only goal right now is to get into your bed. We know you can get there. Because the alternative is waking up in the middle of the night, confused, with a crick in your neck and a sinking feeling that you should have just gotten up and gone to bed in the first place. Then Newton wins, and nobody wants that.

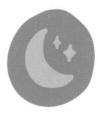

FOR WHEN YOU JUST REMEMBERED SOMETHING REALLY EMBARRASSING YOU SAID YEARS AGO

There are three certainties in life: death, taxes, and being utterly and totally blindsided by the memory of something really embarrassing you said years ago. The first two are mysterious, confusing, and probably best handled by professionals. Unfortunately, that leaves you to deal with the embarrassing memory on your own.

However you behaved in that moment, you're still a good person. Whatever you did—whether you were kind of a bully or you dug your heels in on what turned out to be a bad opinion or you just attempted to say a word out loud that you'd only seen written down (why would they spell *colonel* like that???)—we promise it's okay now. You didn't commit a crime against humanity. Worst-case scenario, it was more like a cringe against humanity, and the International Criminal Court hasn't handed down a life sentence for that offense since the mid-nineties.

Here's the thing: the reason you're embarrassed is because you've grown since then. A large part of why you're such a kind, caring person is because you've learned from all those embarrassing moments that you've had along the way. Have empathy for your past self, even if that past self handled social situations like a baby giraffe trying to learn to walk: awkwardly and with gangly, oversized limbs flying everywhere.

Embarrassing moments—much like milk, eggs and celebrity PR relationships—have an expiration date. We guarantee everyone's already forgotten about whatever you're currently fixating on—up until now, even *you* had forgotten about it!

So file those mortifying memories back to the deep recesses of your brain (nestled in between the Baby Bottle Pop jingle and your childhood best friend's old home phone number) and get on with your day.

You've come too far and achieved too much to dwell on something dumb you said back in seventh grade.

FOR WHEN YOU PROBABLY SHOULD DO SOME KIND OF EXERCISE

Look, we're all mature enough to admit it: everything about exercising kind of sucks.

The digging through your drawers (or laundry pile) to find your cleanest pair of gym shorts. The supportive but deeply heinous shoes. The fact that every piece of equipment you're going to use has been touched by a sweaty person (even if that person was you). We get why you don't want to do it!

But it's the aftermath of the workout that makes it all worthwhile. The flood of endorphins! The excuse to treat yourself to that $14.50 peanut butter protein shake! The ability to casually mention your workout in every conversation tomorrow! It makes sense why people do this every day!

Don't worry about becoming a bodybuilding, marathon-running, spandex-wearing Zumba instructor overnight—in fact, you never have to be any of those things! But if your gut told you to get moving today, then any type of movement is worthwhile. (Doing "The Cupid Shuffle" during a commercial break totally counts.)

So lace up those heinous shoes and get going.

FOR WHEN YOU CAN'T STOP CHECKING WEBMD

A Haiku

Head hurts. Stomach's "off."
Stop searching all your symptoms.
You're fine. We promise.

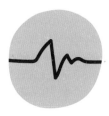

FOR WHEN IT'S TIME TO DO YOUR TAXES (TINY CODDLED BABY EDITION)

gentle harp strum

Well, well, well, if isn't the world's sweetest, gentlest baby-faced angel! Shhh, no, don't get up, you need your rest.

Look, you little dandelion, we totally get it. Taxes are *so* boring and *so* hard. And it's not fair that you *ever* have to do boring and hard things. You're meant to spend your time hugging your friends and gorging yourself on decadent desserts and dancing in fields and playing with dogs. Anything else is simply unfair to you!

But we promise you're going to feel so much better when your taxes are all done. You don't even have to worry about the cents, just round to the nearest dollar. The government could never be mad at you—not with a face like that!

So whenever you have time, maybe just lift your delicate, perfect fingers and finish this silly little task for the silly little government. They'll be thankful, and you'll feel so much better.

FOR WHEN IT'S TIME TO DO YOUR TAXES (TOUGH LOVE EDITION)

SICK GUITAR RIFF

WELL, WELL, WELL, IF IT ISN'T THE KING OF BULLSHIT MOUNTAIN, SITTING ON THEIR THRONE OF NOT DOING THEIR GODDAMN TAXES. WHAT THE ACTUAL FUCK ARE YOU WAITING FOR?

OH, YOU THINK IT'S GOING TO BE BORING? OHHH, YOU THINK IT'S GOING TO BE HARD?? WELL, NEWS FLASH, BUTTERCUP: MOST THINGS ARE BORING AND HARD!! BUT WE HAVE TO DO THEM ANYWAY, SO QUIT YOUR BELLYACHING AND JUST GET 'EM DONE!!!

WHAT'S YOUR PLAN HERE, YOU DIME-STORE SCROOGE MCDUCK? YOU DON'T DO THEM? AND THEN WHAT? YOU SPEND THE REST OF YOUR LIFE AS A FUGITIVE, CONSTANTLY LOOKING OVER YOUR SHOULDER FOR THE IRS?!? IF YOU CAN'T EVEN BRING YOURSELF TO SPEND AN HOUR ENTERING YOUR STUPID LITTLE INCOME INTO A STUPID LITTLE ONLINE FORM, WE PROMISE THAT YOU WILL ABSOLUTELY NOT FARE WELL IN WHITE COLLAR PRISON, DUMBASS!!

JUST DO YOUR TAXES!! OH GOD!! DO IT!!

FOR WHEN YOUR FAVORITE TV SHOW HAS JUST BEEN CANCELED

An Obituary

YOUR FAVORITE TV SHOW
(The Year It Started–The Year It Ended)

Your Favorite TV Show was canceled this week, taken from this world too soon—as the best shows often are—by unforgiving, know-nothing entertainment executives who wouldn't know good television if it ran them over with their own yacht.

Much like generations of television before it, *Your Favorite TV Show* enjoyed the simple things: being on air, having a production budget, and continuing to make new seasons.

While saying goodbye is never easy, this instance is made even more complicated by the fact that none of these characters actually exist, the situations they found themselves in didn't really happen, and you—the show's number one fan—never technically met any of them.

And yet, the loss you're feeling is very real.

How do you say goodbye to a world you've invested so much in? You and *Your Favorite TV Show* have spent hours together. You've been with the characters through their highest highs and lowest lows, you've skipped plans to stay in and watch, you've bruised your thumb fast-forwarding through the intro. You're grieving its loss in a very real way, and that's okay. It's left a butt-shaped imprint on your couch and on your heart.

May its memory live on in reruns forever.

Your Favorite TV Show is predeceased by every other television show that's no longer on the air. It is survived by legions of adoring fans and—God willing—a reboot (or at least a mediocre direct-to-streaming movie) a few years down the road.

In lieu of flowers, please send recommendations for new shows.

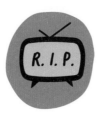

FOR WHEN YOU WANT TO ORDER DELIVERY BUT SHOULD COOK

Quick! We don't have a lot of time before you abandon all plans to cook tonight and order that overpriced gourmet burger, so we've got to work fast. Eyes on us. (We can't actually check that you're doing this, unless you paid for the $5,000 Premium Future-Tech Edition of this book that tracks heat maps of all your eye movements. We're just going to have to trust each other on this.)

First, don't get anywhere near your phone. Throw it across the room if you have to. Your phone is a portal to every restaurant in a ten-mile radius, and they're all waiting and ready to send you food with the click of a button. (Plus a $7.99 delivery fee.)

Next, open your fridge. (Presumably with the hand not holding this book, unless you splurged on the fancy version that levitates.) Take it all in. It's okay if there's not a lot of food in there, or it's mostly just gourmet hot sauces. For example, maybe Past You thought radishes were a good idea, so here we are, staring at a crisper drawer chockablock with radishes. But now you know you have a dozen radishes and most of a bottle of something called Uncle Ron's Certified Near-Death Ghost Pepper Experience. That's a start! (Or maybe an end.)

Before you opened the fridge, you had to choose

between every recipe ever created. That's too big a choice for a Wednesday night! Of course you'd rather get delivery! But now that you've been reacquainted to these radishes? You've got something to work with. You're no longer burdened by the curse of unlimited choice.

Next, go ahead and google "recipes that use radishes," or go analog by grabbing a cookbook off your shelf, blowing off the accumulated dust we assume has gathered, and finding radish in the index. Once you find a recipe that seems moderately appetizing, get to chopping.

Just like that, you've saved $19. Now get cooking! (Unless, of course, you bought the premium edition of this book, which, as we all know, will cook dinner for you.)

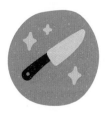

FOR WHEN YOUR HOME IS (REALLY, REALLY) MESSY AND PEOPLE ARE COMING OVER

A Pop Quiz

There's something kind of thrilling about a (really, really) messy house. The adventure of hunting through the clutter for your car keys! The revelation of moving a pile of dirty laundry only to find a shirt you thought you lost months ago! The whimsy of constructing castles out of the dust you found underneath your couch! It's like living in your very own Indiana Jones movie, but without the ancient relics, snakes, or Nazis.

But with that comes the (really, really) terrifying moment when you receive a phone call that someone you know is popping by for a quick visit—a challenge that would make even Indy tremble in his boots.

Before you start furiously cleaning, take a deep breath and use this handy-dandy pop quiz to determine if these unexpected visitors are worth cleaning for.

1. Whoops and/or Woo-hoo! Something really bad/ really good just happened to you. How soon would you tell the people who are coming over?

A) You're on the phone with them *as it's happening.* Or, at the very least, they're one of your very first phone calls after it happens.

B) You'll tell them one of these days! Probably! Maybe! If it comes up!

C) You'd rather chug a whole bottle of spoiled Clamato than tell these people a single thing about yourself.

D) There's nobody coming over, so this question is moot.

2. Quick! Tell us everyone's birthdays and middle names and favorite colors!

A) January 27! Carol! Orangish-reddish!

B) Fall-ish . . . Something with a K, maybe . . . I wanna say blue?

C) Honestly you'd rather not know—it will just rile you up.

D) There's nobody coming over, why do you keep asking me that?

3. What song reminds you of the people coming over?

A) The sound of a child's laughter. The whisper of the wind in the flowers on the first day of spring. Whenever there's beauty in the world, I think of them.

B) Is there a song about casual acquaintances? Because, if so, probably that one.

C) Imagine a movie where Michael Myers, Dracula, and your high school bully all team up. It's whatever the terrifying soundtrack would be.

D) Nobody's coming over!!! Stop it!!!! I mean it!!!!

RESULTS

Mostly As

The people coming over are among your nearest and dearest. You don't have to worry about cleaning for them because they don't care if your house is messy—they're too busy thinking about how great you are. (Or, if they *do* notice the mountain of dishes in your sink, they won't hold it against you.)

Mostly Bs

You barely know the people coming over, which *also* means you shouldn't ruin a perfectly good day frantically scrubbing your floors for loose acquaintances. Instead, offer to meet them in a public place, preferably one with a whole cleaning crew of its own.

Mostly Cs

Friend, it's possible you don't actually like the people that are coming over. Not only should you definitely not clean for them, but you should probably think of an excuse why you can't see them at all. (May we suggest telling them you're "too busy cleaning"?)

Mostly Ds

It doesn't seem like you have anyone coming over, but we admire your surly attitude. Mind if we swing by later?

FOR WHEN YOU'VE HAD WAY TOO MUCH COFFEE

YOU CHUGGED A COFFEE AT 3 PM AND NOW YOUR ONE-WAY TRAIN TO JITTERSTOWN IS LEAVING THE STATION. CHOO-EFFING-CHOO!

Hold on tight, because this train is running express. But don't worry, we're gonna get through this together. When's the last time you took a deep breath?

HUGE BREATH IN

Good, that's the first step. Now blink. Doesn't that feel good? See how casual you are? You definitely still look like a normal human being. No one knows that your insides feel like a volcano and your brain feels like one of those balls of electricity at the science museum.

You *know* that an afternoon cold brew never works out in your favor. But for some reason you thought that maybe today you'd discover you're the Evel Knievel of caffeinated beverage drinkers, astounding everyone with your unbelievable feats of coffee (and also motorcycle stunts). But tough luck, kiddo: turns out you have the same garden-variety body chemistry you always did.

How's about taking another big breath, just like a regular ol' average human would?

ANOTHER HUGE BREATH IN

Nailed it!

We promise this feeling won't last forever—it probably won't even last for the next hour! This caffeine train is eventually going to get to the end of the line, and your life (and heart rate) will go back to normal.

(And if not, maybe just double down and have another coffee. The only way out is through!)

*ONE MORE ENORMOUS BREATH
FOR GOOD MEASURE*

All aboard!

FOR WHEN YOUR CLOTHES DON'T FIT

Okay. So your old clothes aren't fitting you.

Bear with us, because we're going to say a thing that you already know (but that doesn't make it any less important to hear):

They're just clothes. That's it! They're just clothes.

You know what the world is full of? Discount mattress stores. New and improved laundry detergents. Acoustic covers of "Fast Car" by Tracy Chapman. And also articles of clothing. So, so many articles of clothing—including ones that will fit you comfortably, are going to make you feel good, and won't bum you out when you try to wear them. And you deserve to find those.

Think about how much you've experienced since you bought your old clothes. The things you've learned, the trips you've taken, the trashy British dating shows you've binged. You've changed and—naturally—your body has, too. (And thank goodness bodies *do* change, otherwise we'd all still be walking around with the slumping shoulders and raging BO of our middle-school selves.) You're not static, emotionally or physically. No one is. That's why nobody has ever said the words "And the best thing about them? They've worn the same size of jeans since puberty!"

These old clothes have served you well, but now it's time to stick them into the donation pile (or at the very least, into the depths of your closet), where they're not serving as a daily reminder of the size you arbitrarily think you should still be.

And then you're going to go out and enjoy your life in clothes that reflect the vibrant, exciting, magnetic person you are and always have been.

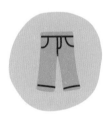

FOR WHEN YOUR HOUSEPLANTS ARE DYING OF THIRST

Just because you forgot to water your plants, that doesn't mean you're a monster.

And just because you planned on watering them but then immediately got distracted, that doesn't mean you are a criminal incapable of taking care of a living thing.

And just because you spent 80 bucks at Lowe's on "kill-proof, low-sun-exposure plants" that you have now singlehandedly ushered to death's door, that doesn't mean you will turn everything you touch to garbage, like some sort of chlorophyll-centric angel of death.

And just because you're currently reading this book, that doesn't mean it's too late to go and water the damn plants right this second.

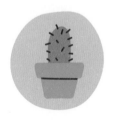

FOR WHEN YOU WANT TO LEAVE THE DIRTY DISHES FOR TOMORROW

A Permission Slip

We, the authors of *Tiny Pep Talks*, hereby give permission to [INSERT NAME HERE] to go ahead and leave the dirty dishes in the sink on the night of [INSERT DATE HERE].

We and our reader, [INSERT NAME HERE], accept the risks associated with this action, which include, but are not limited to: crusty plates, funky smells, and a deep feeling of panic if an unexpected guest shows up before the dishwashing can be completed.

We acknowledge that, okay fine, maybe the "adult" thing to do is to just take three (3) minutes to wash those dang plates. But we also know that life is ultimately a never-ending cycle of dirty dishes and soapy hands, and sometimes you just need a break. So go ahead and take the night off—it's okay with us (this time).*

Warmest regards,
The authors of this book

---

* Please note that this permission slip is null and void if you have roommates. Then you're on your own, kid.

FOR WHEN IT'S TERRIBLE OUTSIDE BUT YOUR DOG NEEDS TO PEE

We hate to say it, friend, but you signed up for this.

There's lots of pets that don't need your supervision to relieve themselves. Cats pee in a box indoors. Horses are presumably already outside. And we're pretty sure snakes don't need to go anywhere special to take a leak (though it's not clear *how* they pee, and we refuse to learn, thank you very much).

But no, you *had* to have a dog, didn't you? And that means you're as committed to the cause as a veteran postal service worker—neither snow nor rain nor heat nor gloom of night will stop these canines from needing to visit the piss palace.

We all know what's going to happen. Ol' Fido is going to be so excited when you grab the leash. And then, when you open the door, he'll realize it's terrible out there. He'll look up at you with those big, watery eyes and wordlessly ask, "Us? Out *there*? Must we?" like it was *your* idea to go outside in the first place.

But as much as you both don't want to leave your warm, dry, IKEA-furnished home, you're gonna march into that storm together. Why? Because your dog is worth it. (And also because otherwise they'll pee all over your POÄNG chair.)

At the end of the (very wet) day, going out in terrible weather is a small price to pay for what you're getting out of this relationship. In return for being present (and making direct and unflinching eye contact) during all of their bowel movements, you're getting constant unconditional love from an extremely photogenic and hilariously eager best friend. Plus, unlike human best friends, your dog is (presumably) never going to ask for the complicated stuff, like lending them money or asking your opinion on their current romantic partner or questioning if this haircut looks good on them. Soggy shoes aside, that's a great deal!

So get out there—together—and know that even if you both come back sopping wet, this is so much better than having to worry about how a snake might pee. (Is it from the tail???)

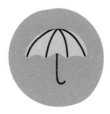

FOR WHEN YOU WOKE UP AT 2 AM AND CAN'T FALL BACK TO SLEEP

A Lullaby

Sung to the tune of "Hush, Little Baby"

Hush, little baby, don't you weep,
It's 2 AM and you can't fall asleep.

Your brain's a mess and your thoughts won't stop,
So we're gonna give you a little pep talk.

You'll fall back asleep, we believe in you!
As long as you do what we tell you to.

Don't look at the clock, don't do the math,
Calculating sleep like a psychopath.

Stop tossing and turning, get out of bed!
You might as well do something else instead.

Go change your spot to a cozy nook,
And we're gonna give you a boring book.

And if that book doesn't make you yawn,
Do a meditation before the dawn.

And if your mind's still not at rest,
Maybe take a quick personality test.

But if that test gives lame results,
Read articles on a few weird cults.

And if that scares you to your bones,
Authors gonna take away your phone.

Wait, why were you on your phone at night?
That's bad for you! No more blue light!

Put that phone across the room,
You'll fall back asleep, we promise you.

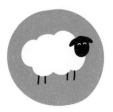

YOU IN THE WORLD

Woo-hoo! You did it!
You left your home! Way to go!
So . . . now what? Don't worry,
we've got your back.

FOR WHEN YOU'RE ABOUT TO SING KARAOKE

Do you remember that headline we all read a few years ago? The one that said public speaking is the most common fear?

Well, if that's true (and it honestly shouldn't be, because a shark with machetes instead of fins is way scarier), then publicly singing a widely beloved song into a microphone—the thing that you're about to do—makes you a gosh darn superhero. We are so proud of you!

So before you go up there, here's what we want you to do:

1. Take a deep breath.

2. Release the tension in your shoulders.

3. Remember that absolutely nobody gives even one iota of a crap how well you do, and frankly they're never going to think about this again.

Seriously, when's the last time you were walking down the street and stopped in your tracks to think, "Hmm, that girl who sang 'Goodbye Earl' at the O'Malley's Pub karaoke night in 2017 sure did a mediocre job!"?

Embarrassment simply has no place at karaoke, and neither does pride. Nobody really cares how well you sing or if you hit the high note or if it turns out you actually *don't* know the third verse of "Rapper's Delight." (Which, for future reference, starts with, "I said I can't wait 'til the end of the week / When I'm rappin' to the rhythm of a groovy beat.")

There are really only two scenarios that could possibly happen when you take the stage:

1. The people listening will think, "Wow! I know this song! Should I get another drink?"

2. The people listening will think, "Wow! I don't know this song! Should I get another drink?"

That's it. End of list. They may tell you "Good job!" or "Nice!" when you get offstage, but they don't actually care. They're probably busy thinking about their own performance, or—if they're smart—they're planning their getaway should they ever encounter Machete Shark.

Break a leg!

FOR WHEN YOU HAVE TO MAKE THAT APPOINTMENT YOU'VE BEEN PUTTING OFF FOR MONTHS

You know what everybody on Earth has in common? (And please don't say something cliché like "innate goodness.")

It's that we're all walking around with a nagging feeling about that appointment we really should have made months ago, whether it's for the dentist, the podiatrist, the accountant, the hair stylist, or some sort of overpriced hybrid of all of the above. (And mention you saw this ad for 10 percent off your next cleaning/bunion shave/tax return/bang trim at Big Earl's One-Stop Clinic!)

But today is the day that you become even better than everybody else, because today is the day that you're making that appointment.

Look, we won't lie to you. The five minutes that the call is going to take might suck. It could be awkward, you'll probably have to talk to a stranger, and you'll definitely have to look at your calendar. None of these things are fun. There's a reason that Disney World never opened that "Getting on the Phone and Making Appointments" section of the park. (But can we agree that Mickey's Wild Copay Roller Coaster would have been *awesome*?)

But it's the feeling *after* the call that's going to make it all worthwhile. It's like a runner's high without all the chafing. No matter what else you do today, you'll have crossed something big off your to-do list. You'll have done Future You a favor. And wow, you'll have definitely earned an afternoon off from worrying about all those other appointments you still have to make.

Get to dialing!

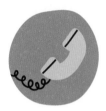

FOR WHEN YOU HAVE TO PARALLEL PARK

Beep, beep!

Look who it is: the best driver in the world!

In fact, you are *so* good at driving that the government got together and gave you a cute little card granting you permission to drive a two-ton steel machine around at 65 miles per hour. Look at you go!

We get it. Parallel parking *is* hard. Cars just weren't meant to go sideways. But you've made it this far. Take a deep breath, adjust the rearview mirror, and take your time. Nobody is judging you. We've all been there.

Plus, if you bump into the car behind you a little bit, is it really *that* big a deal? If they *really* cared about their car, they shouldn't be parking it on the street for anyone to hit, so that's kind of on them.

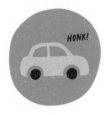

FOR WHEN YOU LEFT LATE
AND NOW THERE'S TRAFFIC

You sweet, naive prodigy of procrastination. We hope you're ready, because here's the cold, hard truth.

Unless your dashboard is equipped with some sort of supersonic, aerospace-grade, ultra-high-powered turbo booster lever, you're probably gonna be late. The sooner you realize that, the easier this is all going to be. There's no use fighting it or beating yourself up about it—you barely have enough time as it is.

The good news is the people at your destination will understand, because—much like tummy aches and being swindled by a shrewd telemarketer—traffic is one of those universal excuses. Plus patience is famously a virtue, so ultimately, waiting for you is good for their character. You're actually doing *them* a huge favor!

You'll get there when you get there.

FOR WHEN YOU AGREED TO SOMETHING MONTHS AGO AND NOW IT'S TIME TO ACTUALLY DO IT

You gotta give it up for Past You—that bastard really grabbed life by the horns.

The poet Mary Oliver once asked, "Tell me, what is it you plan to do with your one wild and precious life?" And Past You responded with a resounding, "EVERYTHING, ACTUALLY," their eyes glazed, fingers flying, as they accepted evite after evite for events months down the road.

But Current You? Current You could not be more different. You've grown, you've changed, you've come to realize what really matters to you! And, it turns out, what really matters is quietly sitting at home, keeping to yourself, and staying far, far away from social situations.

Current You has two options:

1. You can just bail! It's fine! Cancel your plans, hoist your sweatpants up as high as they'll go, microwave a plate full of pizza bagels, and check in for the night. That's okay! (For the record, we're assuming here that the plans in question are something like going to dinner with your downstairs neighbor and fourteen of their cousins, not

something important like officiating a wedding or helping a friend get out of some light tax-fraud charges.)

2. Consider if maybe . . . just maybe . . . Past You had a good point. Perhaps that son of a bitch and their adventurous spirit had it all figured out. Maybe the reason that the plans in question sounded fun to you back then was because Past You knew you'd have a good time. Sure, it's way easier to do the same thing night after night—but sometimes, it's worth being uncomfortable for a few minutes in order to have nights worth remembering.

The best thing to do—as Current You, in this current moment—is to look out for Future You. What's going to be best for them? Is it to stay in, get some rest, and catch up on your shows? (Sometimes the answer is going to be yes!) Or is it to go out and have fun? (Sometimes the answer will be a resounding yes to that one, too.)

Whatever you choose, Future You will be thankful.

FOR WHEN YOU'RE OVERDRESSED

Hey there, knockoff Jay Gatsby. So you've misinterpreted the "semiformal streetwear meets 1800s Paris" dress code, and you've arrived completely overdressed.

It's okay! At the end of the day, your problem is that you're the most glamorous guest here, which is a pretty cool thing to be. So don't run off just yet to weep to your chauffeur from the back of your 1933 drop-top Rolls-Royce!

First, is there anything you can do to change up your look to feel a bit more casual? Maybe take off that Komodo dragon skin coat? Remove a few of the larger diamonds? Go outside and rub a little dirt on your tuxedo? There. Much better.

Second, understand that there's really nothing else you can do but lean into this. Keep asking about the vintage of the box of Franzia. Politely refuse to try the Domino's pizza because "once you've had the real thing, you can't go back." Confuse everyone by slipping a crisp five-dollar bill into the pocket of the host. Remember: you're not *overdressed*, they're all *underdressed*!

And hey, it could be worse. You could be dressed like one of the side characters from the Country Bear Jamboree.

FOR WHEN YOU'RE UNDERDRESSED

Well, well, well, if it isn't one of the side characters from the Country Bear Jamboree. So you misinterpreted the "funky cocktail chic meets '90s Phoenix, Arizona" dress code, and you've arrived completely underdressed.

Remove that piece of straw you've been chewing on and repeat after us: it's fine. So you're underdressed for an event? Big whoop! You know who else underdresses for events? Rock stars. Celebrity chefs. Billionaires cosplaying as normal people. So don't run off just yet to blast Lynyrd Skynyrd in your 1976 Ford Gran Torino.

First, is there anything you can do to gussy up your outfit just a smidge? Can you tuck in your shirt? (If you haven't put on a shirt, do that first.) Is there anything you can use to help keep up your jorts? If no one else is playing Edward 40 Hands, maybe consider un-taping the malt liquor from your fists? There. Much better.

Second, understand that there's nothing left to do but bring Fun Uncle Energy™ to this party. Challenge other guests to arm wrestle. Come up with a catchphrase and use it liberally. Strike up a conversation about how fast NASCAR goes. (Spoiler: it goes so fast.) Remember: you're not underdressed, they're all overdressed!

And hey, it could be worse. You could be dressed like a knockoff Jay Gatsby.

FOR WHEN YOU'RE ON HOUR SIX OF AN EIGHT-HOUR DRIVE

It was Willie Nelson who once said, "On the road again / Just as long as it's not more than three hours or so / Any more than that's too much / But other than that / I just can't wait to get on the road again." (We're paraphrasing here, but that's the gist of it.)

But once again, you went against the Word of Willie, because here you are on hour six of an eight-hour road trip. And you don't know how much more you can take.

Here's the thing, buddy: there's nothing left to do but keep going forward. (Right now, we're talking about your road trip, but feel free to apply that to anything else happening in your life.)

What are you going to do, stop at the next town you pass and start a new life there with nothing but your car, the pack of mints in the center console, and a couple of empty coffee cups that were rolling around in the back seat? Change your name to The Deuce, grow your hair long, and get a job at the old mill? Find a nice townsperson to settle down with, get a dog, a cat, maybe a few kids, and live out the rest of your days content in a way you previously never thought possible?

Nope. Sorry. As tempting as that may be, that's not you, buddy.

So instead, you're going to pull over at the next gas station. You're going to get yourself your favorite road trip snack—the more sodium the better—and you're going to fire up some deep cuts on the ol' playlist. It's going to be long. It's going to be boring. But it's already *been* long and boring—the difference now is that you'll get there that much sooner.

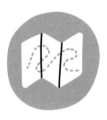

FOR WHEN YOU'RE ABOUT TO LEAVE FOR A BIG TRIP

An In-Flight Announcement

PA system crackles on

Welcome to Tiny Pep Air, these are your captains speaking. We just got word from air traffic control that you're about to be cleared to take off on a big trip. But before you leave, we have a few quick in-flight announcements.

It looks like it'll be mostly smooth flying all the way to your destination. But even if we hit a few bumps—and with travel, there's always a *few* bumps—it's nothing you can't handle. Every trip has some unexpected turbulence along the way.

Before we take off, all phones and large electronic devices need to be stowed and turned to airplane mode. Wait, actually, why don't you just turn those all off right now. There's no need to look up statistics on plane malfunctions or what's really up with the in-flight meals. You're taking a trip to relax, not to give your anxiety something new to focus on.

If at any point in the trip we experience a change in cabin pressure—and by that we mean you start putting too much pressure on this trip to be "amazing" or "life-changing" or "the best trip anyone's ever had in the history of travel"—a hand will drop from the ceiling to slap you out of it. (Okay, not really, but don't do that. Giving yourself unrealistic expectations sets you up for disappointment.)

When we arrive at your destination, your luggage will be waiting for you. But if you find that you've forgotten something you meant to pack—or if your bag ended up on a different flight entirely—remember that stores still exist in almost every other place, and you'll be able to get what you need. (And do you really need to brush your teeth *every* day anyway?)

Before we take off, two last reminders: (1) the fasten seatbelt sign is on, and (2) we're proud of you for taking this trip. You deserve it. No matter how much planning, organization, and deep breaths into a paper bag it took, you're here now. So sit back, relax, and enjoy your flight on Tiny Pep Air.

Flight crew, prepare the cabin for takeoff.

FOR WHEN YOU'RE
AWKWARDLY EARLY

They say the early bird gets the worm, but you arrived early and all you got was an awkward amount of time on your hands. (Not that a worm sounds particularly delicious, either.)

Maybe you hit every green light on the way here. Maybe your friend who's perpetually late tricked you into believing that, for once, they would actually be on time. Or maybe you just checked in for your 4 PM appointment and it's only 10:10 AM. (You wanted to be safe!)

There's no shame in being early. If you did anything wrong (which you didn't), it was caring too much. You prioritized this obligation above all else, which is a very kind thing to do. That pretty much makes you the patron saint of not wasting people's time!

Patience is a virtue and you deserve to be rewarded for yours. Go grab a snack, embark on a small adventure, or draw doodles on this page. Do whatever sounds fun, just don't sit and twiddle your thumbs. (Unless twiddling is your thing, in which case, twiddle away, dude!)

There's not a lot of constants in this world, but one is that time moves ever forward. So as awkward as it might feel right now to be early, we promise—with complete certainty—that you'll be on time very soon.

FOR WHEN YOUR PHONE BATTERY IS AT 5 PERCENT

Brace yourself: your phone's about to die.

It's up to you: you can either totally interrupt your day by hunting down a charger (and an outlet . . . and a place to sit while you charge it . . .), or you can spend your last gasp of battery life playing Bejeweled, secure in the knowledge that if the *Seinfeld* gang could get through nearly nine seasons without a cell phone, you can definitely make it through the rest of your day.

Just remember this one crucial thing: **if you really need—**

phone dies

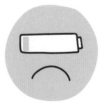

FOR WHEN YOU'RE REALLY BAD AT SOMETHING THAT YOU'VE NEVER TRIED BEFORE

A Very Sarcastic Pep Talk

WOWIE ZOWIE! So you tried something you've never done before and you were really bad at it?! Color us shocked![1]

Being bad at something that you've never tried before is the worst possible scenario that could ever happen to anyone.[2] Ever.[3] This whole situation must be really devastating for you.[4] We don't know how you'll ever recover.[5]

---

[1] We are neither wowied nor zowied about this fact at all. Don't color us shocked! If anything, color us more of an unfazed shade of Crayola Manatee Gray!

[2] False. The worst possible scenario that could ever happen to anyone is realizing it's the last day of school and you have to pass the big final to graduate, but you haven't been to class all semester, and this time it is not a dream, it's very real, and also you're naked for some reason.

[3] Or maybe the worst scenario is the same as above, but also it's opening night of the big play you're starring in and you don't know any of your lines. (And you're still super naked.)

[4] We love you, you're literally the best, but this isn't devastating. It honestly would have been weird if you were amazing at something on your first try.

[5] This is going to be funny by next week, if not by tomorrow.

People spend literal years honing their craft, but it totally makes sense that you thought you'd be able to do it perfectly on your first try.[6] You're different![7] You're better![8] The rules for other people don't apply to you![9]

One thing is for sure: everyone you know is going to find out about this,[10] and they'll be disappointed and frankly appalled that you were bad at something you've never tried before.[11] This is all they're going to be talking about for *weeks*—months, even.[12] They've certainly never been bad at anything new before,[13] so this is understandably going to change the way they see you, permanently.[14]

No matter what happens, don't try again.[15] What if you're bad at something the second time you do it?![16]

---

[6] Nobody is an expert at something the first time they try it, except those spooky little five-year-olds that came out of the womb knowing how to play Tchaikovsky on violin.

[7] You *are* different!

[8] You *are* better!

[9] But that doesn't change the fact that some rules, laws, and basic scientific theories—including this one—still apply to you.

[10] They won't. There's no trade publication called *People Doing Things Kinda Badly Their First Time*.

[11] Nobody's going to think twice about this. They're all too busy thinking about a meme they saw earlier.

[12] Seriously, they're not going to remember this in an hour.

[13] Yes, they have been.

[14] If anything, they may see you as someone cooler and more willing to try something new! An inspiration, really!

[15] If you had fun and/or are contractually obligated to try it again, go for it!

[16] You probably will be! And that's okay!

YOU & OTHER PEOPLE:
STRANGERS & ACQUAINTANCES

There's a reason the TOY STORY producers scrapped their song "You've Got a Casual Acquaintance in Me." While people you kinda know can be great, they can also be a Minesweeper board of sticky situations. We're here to help.

FOR WHEN YOU'RE GOING TO A PARTY AND YOU ONLY KNOW ONE PERSON

Maybe going to a party where you only know one person is your dream, you majestic social butterfly. But maybe you're planning to strategically position yourself next to the chip bowl all night so that instead of making small talk, you can spend a few hours anxiously stuffing fistfuls of Harvest Cheddar Sun Chips into your mouth. While that's honestly not a bad strategy, you deserve better.

First off, can we say: you look great. That outfit? On point. Your hair? In its ideal form. Your scent? Inoffensive. If we were at this party, we'd be psyched to get to meet you. And we bet everyone else is going to feel that way, too.

Before you walk in, remember that whoever invited you to this party must really like you, and they think everyone else is going to like you, too. People don't get invited to parties by accident—they get invited because they're smart, funny, and interesting. And that's you, baby!

The worst-case scenario is that you're going to spend a couple of hours being nice to some strangers. You're gonna have to nod politely at some lame jokes, you're gonna have to answer the question "Sooo . . . what do

68

you do?" thirty times, and you're gonna sneak into the bathroom at least once just to sit and silently scroll on your phone. That all adds up to a perfectly fine night and, honestly, like 80 percent of all experiences are just that anyway—perfectly fine!

The best-case scenario—and this is the one that we're secretly sure will happen—is that you'll charm an entire room full of strangers, who will all be texting each other the next day saying, "I loved meeting that awesome new person last night!" You're like Cinderella, but with the ability to keep track of both your shoes and surrounded by fewer singing rodents. (Probably.)

Wherever you're going and whatever the night holds, you're gonna be great.

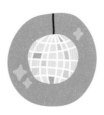

FOR WHEN IT'S TIME TO SPLIT THE BILL

A Mathematical Equation

Quiz time, math whiz!

2 + 2 = 4 (Great, nailed it.)

3 x 3 = 9 (That one was a little harder, but nothing can stop you, brainiac!)

Now what about the dreaded:

"Let's just split it down the middle" ÷ who had the 3 cocktails and why were they $18 each? x your friend's $63 steak frites − (your $12.50 salad + the appetizer you didn't even really eat + tip + tax + something called a "service referendum"?) x anxiety³

As tricky as the math is, you don't have to take out a small business loan just because your dining companion ordered something called "beluga caviar sliders" and now wants to go splitsies. Unless they cleared it with the table (and Greenpeace) beforehand, you shouldn't have to chip in for someone else's extravagance.

Go ahead and speak up if you don't feel comfortable splitting the bill evenly—you'll be the hero this table needs. At the end of the day, you gotta look out for number one. That's just basic math.

FOR WHEN YOU'VE HAD SPINACH IN YOUR TEETH ALL DAY AND NOBODY TOLD YOU

Uh oh . . . there's something in your teeth. And we regret to inform you that that piece of stowaway spinach has been there since lunch and no one said a damn thing.

Maybe you're worried everyone you interacted with today noticed, purposely didn't tell you, and is calling you "Little Lord Spinach Head, Vampire of the Leafy Greens" in their group chats right now.

But they're not. We promise. If somebody had noticed, they would have said something—both because they've got your back and because everyone loves being the person who points out you have something in your teeth. (It makes them feel powerful.)

So, unless you got married today or just finished posing for the centerfold the next issue of *Perfect Teeth Weekly*, this stays between you and that little chewed-up wad of spinach.

FOR WHEN SOMEBODY SPOILS YOUR FAVORITE SHOW

History is filled with some pretty terrible people. Vlad the Impaler. Jack the Ripper. And now Your Friend the Show Spoiler.

Whatever TV show they just spoiled for you (just spitballing here, but we're guessing it's one about rich people with dark secrets making bad decisions), there's no excuse for that kind of behavior. You have a life. You can't be expected to drop everything and watch a show the moment it comes out! This is an atrocity.

But as hard as this may be, what are you going to do? Stop watching? Here's a spoiler alert for you, buddy: you can still love the show, even though you sort of know what's going to happen. The thing is, you don't watch a show just for the ending. It's all about the way it unfolds. (And also about the weird little crush you develop on that one character along the way.)

You're gonna get through this. Just know you can never trust that friend again.

FOR WHEN YOU JUST SPOILED THAT SHOW FOR SOMEONE

Oh, gosh, it's totally fine! Mistakes happen every day. This isn't an atrocity, it's just a television show. Who on Earth could ever stay mad about something like that?

Getting a show spoiled for you is the gamble we take when we don't watch something the moment it comes out. Your friend accepted that risk the second they hit PLAY on a show that came out months ago. If they really cared, they would have already caught up on all the episodes.

Plus, actually, you kind of *helped* them. Nothing's more stressful than the unknown—and by spoiling the show for them, you alleviated some of that anxiety. So in a way, you're kind of a hero, and should go down in history as such.

Alexander the Great. Richard the Lionheart. And You the Compassionate Spoiler of Shows.

FOR WHEN YOU HAVE TO TELL THE SERVER THAT'S NOT WHAT YOU ORDERED

There it is, right in front of you: a perfectly executed Cobb salad. Every one of the 500 ingredients has been plated with care. The greens have the exact right amount of dressing. The eggs are also there for some reason. It's perfectly crafted for you to take the ideal bite.

The problem is, you ordered the burger. And now you're going to have to tell the server.

Look, we get the reasons why you might not want to tell the server they got it wrong. You don't want to seem rude! Sending the food back means you have to wait even longer to eat! Plus maybe the chef will come out from the kitchen, red-faced and sweaty, to tell you off while wildly waving a meat cleaver! It's scary!

But, come on: what would the chef yell and threaten you with a cleaver for? You didn't mess up, you're not going to be rude, and there's zero reason to compromise on this besides your own fear of conflict. If your coworker got your name totally wrong, would you never correct them and just become a new person? No! Unless that name was something really cool, like "T-Bone."

Real talk? The restaurant wants you to have the burger, too. They'd so much rather make it right than have you leave dinner with a bad taste in your mouth. Ultimately, the only person keeping you from chowing down on that delicious burger—a burger that you specifically left the house for—is you.

So politely flag down that server and let them know what's going on. Because you deserve that burger, and somewhere out there, someone else is waiting for their Cobb salad.

FOR WHEN YOU 1,000 PERCENT FORGOT THAT GUY'S NAME

A Sherlock Holmes Mystery

Well, well, well, Sherlock—you've once again fetched up a vexing mystery, this time in "The Case of the Man with the Vanishing Name." We're sure you'll determine this acquaintance's name in no time with your superior powers of deduction!

Enter your mind palace and lay out the clues before you. What do you know that might jog your memory to solve this conundrum?

You know that you follow this chap on Instagram, where he uses the nom de plume GatorDaddy—but that almost certainly cannot be his Christian name.

Scan his face—does he have any unique or discernable features that could help? He has the visage and general vibe of a Dylan . . . is that anything? Have you just found the key that unlocks this puzzle? Think, think! This is usually so elementary!

Don't worry, Holmes. If your genius brain doesn't deduce the answer, then it will surely come up with a clever workaround, such as saying, "Hey, you! Long time no see!" or "You know what would be splendid? Saying our names out loud, just for fun!"

And when you've eliminated the impossible, whatever remains, however improbable, must be the truth. Maybe his name actually *is* GatorDaddy?

The game's afoot!

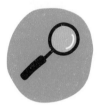

FOR WHEN YOU HAVE A BIG JUICY SECRET THAT YOU ABSOLUTELY CANNOT SHARE UNDER ANY CIRCUMSTANCES

A Loophole

The hardest thing humans have to do—besides unpacking suitcases after big trips and parallel parking in front of a crowded restaurant patio—is to keep a big, juicy, jaw-dropping secret that you absolutely cannot share under any circumstances.

You're doing a great job. You're a responsible human who keeps things to themselves when they are asked to. But even so, isn't the whole fun of having a secret seeing people's reactions when you spill the beans? (Which, we must stress again, you really, really can't do.)

Good news, though! There's a glaring loophole right in front of us. You can't tell any other *person*, sure. But what about telling . . . a book?

Go ahead. Whisper the secret right into the page here. This is a safe space. Who are we going to tell? (And, more importantly, *how* are we—the presumably impossibly hot and charming versions of the authors you have in your head—going to tell?)

*
*
*
*
*
*
*

OH, GOSH. WOW!!!! WE CAN'T BELIEVE IT. WE ARE SO SURPRISED/EXCITED/FLABBER-GASTED/UPSET TO HEAR THAT!!!!!!!!!!!!!! HOLY COW!!!!!!!! OUR JAWS—OR WHATEVER THE BOOK EQUIVALENT IS—ARE ON THE FLOOR, FROM JOY AND/OR SHOCK!!!!!!

This is, undoubtedly, the most amazing secret we have ever heard, and we're impressed with you for knowing it. You are so brave for keeping it inside of you for so long. Thank you for trusting us with this knowledge.

There. Doesn't that feel a little bit better? (Just remember, you seriously cannot tell *anyone* else. This stays between us.)

FOR WHEN YOU'RE THINKING OF TELLING EVERYONE ABOUT A WEIRD DREAM YOU HAD ONCE

A Crossword Puzzle

ACROSS

1. Don't _____ it
2. Don't _____ it
3. Don't _____ it
4. Don't do _____
5. _____ do it
6. _____ do it
7. Don't _____ it
8. Don't do _____
9. Don't do _____

DOWN

1. _____ do it
3. _____ do it
5. Don't _____ it
6. Don't _____ it
8. Don't do _____

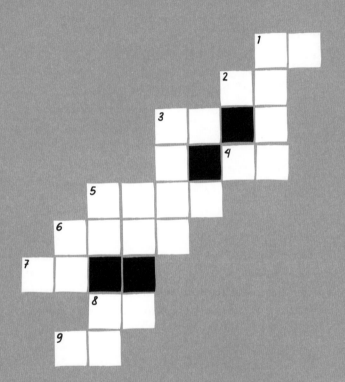

FOR WHEN YOU NEED TO ASK THE NEIGHBORS TO PLEASE, PLEASE, PLEASE KEEP IT DOWN

Willkommen to Klub Neighbor, the hottest club this side of the Brandenburg Gate! Here, the bass is always bumping, the crowd never stops stomping, and there's always an opportunity to randomly scream! The party starts every night at 11 PM and goes until whenever we freaking feel like it!

. . . is the invitation you wish your neighbors had sent you before you moved in. But here we are, once again, sharing walls with the loudest people in the universe. You've got a big day ahead of you tomorrow (it's Tuesday night, folks), so unfortunately, it looks like you're going to need to ask the neighbors to please, please, please keep it down.

Here's the thing: you're the one who's in the right. You're not the fun police coming to school to give a presentation on why homework rules and smoking drools. You're a human being whose needs matter—and what you need right now is for your neighbors to shut the hell up.

Unless they're like Jason Statham's character in the 2006 film *Crank* and they have to keep their heart rate up with loud music and wild parties or else they'll die, it's not an inconvenience to ask them to stop inconveniencing you. And if they *are* like Jason Statham's character in the 2006 film *Crank*, you might want to consider moving.

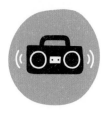

YOU & OTHER PEOPLE:

FRIENDS & FAMILY

Look, of course you love your friends and family! They're the best! Everyone else's friends and families suck in comparison! That's just facts! But that doesn't mean it's all smooth sailing. When things start to get bumpy, you've got us.

FOR WHEN YOUR FRIEND KEEPS SUGGESTING A PODCAST THAT YOU HAVE NO INTEREST IN LISTENING TO

Let's cut to the chase: there's a less than zero percent chance you're going to listen to that podcast your friend keeps suggesting.

We all know you're going to politely say, "It's on my list!" But that's not true—there is no list. There's never been a list. And starting that list would be a huge pain in the you-know-what. The rising cost of paper! Choosing a style of bullet points! Remembering all the other times you've used this lie before! Where would you even begin?!

So, good news: we created that list for you! Now anytime someone suggests a podcast or a TV show or a six-episode docu-special that you sure as shit aren't going to even start, you can honestly say you're "putting it on your list."

_____[YOUR NAME]_____'s

List of Media They Never Intend to Actually Consume

- That one podcast your friend keeps suggesting

- That new show everyone likes, starring that actor, what's-their-face, from that other show everyone likes

- That gruesome murder documentary with dubious investigative practices and a whole lot of bloodlust

- That "seriously life-changing" book suggested by your messiest friend

- That reality show that's been on for twenty-six seasons (that you *have* to start from the beginning)

- *Mad Men*

- _____

- _____

- _____

FOR WHEN YOU'RE GONNA HAVE TO SEE THAT ONE COUSIN

Sung to the tune of "Santa Claus Is Coming to Town"

You better watch out,
You better not cry,
You better not pout,
I'm telling you why,
That one cousin's coming to town.

He's making a list,
Of all of this thoughts;
He's sharing his opinions if you want 'em or not.
That one cousin's coming to town.

He wears shorts in the winter,
He always shows up late.
His parents say, "He's gonna change!"
But this year he's thirty-eight.

Oh!

You better watch out,
You better not scream,
You better not ask
'Bout his new get-rich scheme.
That one cousin's coming to town.

You only have to see him
A couple times a year,
So if he gets to be too much,
Your phone is always near!

Oh!

You better watch out.
No shame in a break!
There's no need to please
A grown man who loves snakes.
That guy's got a room full of snakes.

FOR WHEN YOU THINK YOU MIGHT HATE YOUR FRIEND'S PARTNER

Thank God you're here, and not a second too late. Any longer and you might have gone from *thinking* you hate your friend's partner to *knowing* you hate your friend's partner—and that's a waterslide you can't paddle your wet butt back up.[*]

Read this sentence twice if you have to: you cannot, under any circumstances, admit to yourself that you hate your friend's partner.

The moment you take a bite of that particular apple of Eden, it's all over. The world's axis will shift and you will never be able to go back. You'll go from being a chill, carefree person, mostly unfazed by your friend's partner's never-ending stories about the time they studied abroad fifteen years ago, to a dark, spiteful husk of yourself hellbent on undermining them every time they talk.

Ultimately, your friend's relationship is none of your business. Okay, sure, do you wish that their partner were

[*] Important note: This pep talk assumes your friend's partner is exceedingly boring or unlikable but ultimately harmless. If your friend's partner is putting you or your friend in physical or emotional danger, that person is definitely bad. Take any actionable steps you can to help get your friend away from them. You may want to start with consulting an additional, more serious book.

smarter, or more thoughtful, or less of a total bore who you'd push out a twelfth story window without a second thought if it meant you wouldn't have to listen to their inane stories for one more moment? Of course, we've all been there! But it's not your relationship, it's your friend's. And thank goodness for that—if their partner is this annoying at a party, imagine what a nightmare they'd be when kissing's involved.

The best thing to do is support your friend and tolerate their partner. (This is one and only time in this book when we'll advocate for repressing your feelings, so soak it in, kid.)

Awesome. Crisis ignored. And the next time you're trapped listening to one of their never-ending stories that you simply had to be there for, just push those feelings down. For the sake of your friendship!

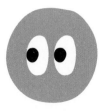

FOR WHEN YOU'RE WORRIED YOUR FRIENDS ARE ALL SECRETLY MAD AT YOU

Your friends aren't mad at you. They never have been and, if they were, someone would have told you by now.

They're just all busy online shopping and paying bills and worrying that *their* friends are all mad at *them*. Like everyone is, all the time.

We promise.

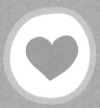

FOR WHEN YOU FORGOT THEIR BIRTHDAY

Dagnabbit! Last night, you drifted to sleep believing yourself to be the Most Thoughtful Person in the World, only to wake up in a cold sweat, haunted by the realization that you fully forgot your friend's/family member's/college roommate's/favorite barista's birthday.

Hey, it happens! Even you—still the Most Thoughtful Person in the World—can't be expected to keep track of every significant date for every person you care about. That doesn't make you a bad person—it just makes you a person who forgot to add this one event to your calendar. (And also maybe a person who got a little too reliant on Facebook notifications to remind you of birthdays.)

Here's the deal: text them, call them, write them a card, send them a carrier pigeon, whatever you want to do—but do it now. Seriously, right now. Harness this guilt for good!

No matter if you're a few hours, a few days, or a few weeks late, we promise that they will be delighted to hear from you (who wouldn't be!), and that delight will outweigh any tardiness in your well wishes. Plus, this way, you're extending their birthday celebrations, which is a gift in itself. (And that's exactly the kind of behavior that makes you the Most Thoughtful Person in the World.)

FOR WHEN YOUR FRIEND IS GOING THROUGH IT AND YOU DON'T KNOW WHAT TO SAY

Unless you're a therapist, a lawyer, or a mob boss granting favors on this, the day of your daughter's wedding, your friend probably didn't share their troubles with you because they want you to fix them. They shared them with you because they love you and want you beside them while they go through it.

And what a privilege it is to hold that position in someone's life.

You don't need to say the perfect thing because there's not a perfect thing to say. There isn't a sentence that, if spoken, will magically make them feel better, ensuring that no bad things happen to them—or to anyone—ever again. (And honestly, even if there were, that's too much responsibility for one person. The world would be banging down your door with sob stories and corporate brand deals.)

All you can do is check in. Be there for them. Tell them you care about them. Give them space to talk about their feelings or to not talk about their feelings. Hoard funny corgi videos to have at the ready, just in case they need a laugh. Send them texts. Bake them cookies. Buy them cookies and take credit for baking them. Call them when you're stuck in traffic just to tell them you're thinking about them. And when there's nothing you can say, all you have to be is the person beside them.

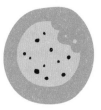

FOR WHEN YOU LEAVE YOUR KID WITH A BABYSITTER FOR THE FIRST TIME

So it's really happening. You're actually leaving your kid with a babysitter for the first time.

It's tempting to play the *Greatest Hits of Everything That Could Go Wrong* on repeat in your head—all your favorites, like "Help! (My Baby's Trapped in the Garbage Disposal)" and "The Babysitter's in a Cult (And Now My Baby Is, Too)" and the unforgettable "Went to One Dinner (And Child Protective Services Came A-Knockin')." But none of that is going to happen tonight.

You're a great parent, and this isn't anything you can't handle. As absurd as it seems to trust a thirteen-year-old to do anything responsible—let alone care for your literal child—you're doing the right thing. You left detailed instructions for bedtime, you triple-checked the sitter has your number, and you hid the good snacks away in the upstairs closet. There's nothing left to do except go to dinner, have a silly little drink, and check your cell phone every thirty seconds (even though you don't have to). And when you get home, your kid will still be there, in one piece and (hopefully) sound asleep.

Everything is gonna be fine.

FOR WHEN YOUR PARENTS LEAVE YOU WITH A BABYSITTER FOR THE FIRST TIME

So it's really happening. Your parents—those traitors, those bamboozlers, those jerks—have abandoned you with the oldest stranger in the world.

We get it, kid. There's a lot of uncertainty here. What if this babysitter doesn't follow your special bedtime routine? What if they're not familiar with Margaret Wise Brown's seminal work *Goodnight Moon*? And God help them if they try to cut your grilled cheese in a way that isn't up to your exacting requirements.

You're a great kid, and this isn't anything you can't handle. Plus, remember that this is your house and not theirs, so see how far you push it: Ice cream sundaes for dinner! Screen time till your eyes water! Bedtime shmedtime, you're partying till 8:30-ish tonight!

And when your parents get home—and they're gonna be home soon—they're gonna be so happy to see you that they won't even care about any of tonight's shenanigans.

Everything is gonna be fine.

FOR WHEN YOU'RE BABYSITTING FOR A FAMILY WHO'S LEAVING THEIR KID FOR THE FIRST TIME

So it's really happening. After, like, thirty minutes of goodbyes and reviewing eight pages of laminated instructions, the parents are finally leaving their kid for the night.

They're acting like no one in the history of time has ever left their kid with a babysitter before. But we can assure you that when cave-parents Grog and Unkh left their baby at home in the year one zillion BC, their sitter certainly hadn't taken an eight-hour babysitting certificate course like you have. Evolutionarily, you're way more prepared than that stupid cave-babysitter!

You're a great babysitter, and this isn't anything you can't handle. Sometimes babysitting means you have to do some parent-sitting, too. You're going to ace responding to the parents' nervous texts, you're going to follow the incredibly detailed bedtime routine to a T, and you're gonna help yourself to all the choice snacks you found hidden in the upstairs closet. No matter how nervous the kid and the parents look now, by the end of the night you're going to be a hero.

Everything is gonna be fine.

FOR WHEN YOUR FRIENDS START HAVING KIDS

Look, it goes without saying that you're happy for your friends. Of course you are! Your friends are going to be amazing parents! The world is better off when kind, compassionate people raise more kind, compassionate people! That kid is probably going to grow up to cure every disease and win a dozen Nobel Prizes, even the boring ones!

But, at the same time, your friends having kids may be bringing up a thousand other feelings for you, too. And that's completely okay.

Maybe this has you worried about your own place in your friend's life. Maybe the idea of parenthood brings up a wave of concern anxiety, grief, and frustration. Maybe you're upset that all your hangouts are going to be crashed by a tiny, sticky stranger who refuses to split the bill.

However you're feeling, it's time for you to take a deep breath and do a little parenting—of yourself. Send yourself to bed early when you're feeling cranky. Put yourself in time-out when you need a little break. Give yourself a treat (or twenty) for working through so many big feelings. And, most importantly, remember that you're doing your best—so treat yourself with patience, forgiveness, and a whole lot of kindness. You deserve it.

FOR WHEN YOU HAVE TO APOLOGIZE

Oopsie daisy, you acted like a big ol' jerk!

It's okay, bud. Despite your best efforts, you're gonna be a jerk sometimes. It's true! We'd never lie to you! *(And if we ever have, we're so sorry!)* Whether it's accidental, on purpose, or just an involuntary impulse brought on by having a measly 7.5 hours of sleep the night before, we're all the villain in the story sometimes. What's important is that you've come to the conclusion that you have to apologize. We're proud of you.

But now comes the tough part: actually saying you're sorry. Apologizing is hard! It can be awkward, it can be upsetting, and it can lead to seriously unfun conversations about the way your actions made other people feel. And we don't blame you if you'd rather have the dentist yank your teeth out with a pair of bargain-bin salad tongs than go through that experience. But ultimately, it's the right thing to do, and it's going to make everyone involved feel better, including you. *(Sorry if that's too forward!) (And sorry for bringing up the dentist earlier!)*

Whatever happened, you're still a good person—that's why you're apologizing in the first place! You know who never apologizes? Power-hungry dictators! Narcissistic millionaires! Masked-up horror movie franchise villains!

(Excluding, of course, Bela Lugosi's classic 1933 film, Dracula Expresses Remorse. But you already knew that. Sorry if it seemed like we were patronizing you!) And you're better than all of those people! *(Sorry if that offends anyone!)* So apologize sincerely and keep moving forward—a little more kind, a little more aware, and a little bit less of a jerk.

You can do it. *(Sorry if we're coming on too strong.)*

FOR WHEN YOU CAN SEE YOUR PARENTS GEARING UP TO HAVE A BIG CONVERSATION BEFORE THE END OF THE VISIT

Uh oh . . . there's a storm a-brewin'. The air is buzzing with anticipation and obvious knowing glances between your parents. You know—you just KNOW—that your parents are going to try to have a Big Conversation with you before the end of the visit.

You're caught in the middle of a field without a raincoat, and Hurricane We-Need-to-Have-a-Chat is bearing down fast.

You've got two options, friend:

You can try to outrun the storm. As long as you keep the small talk moving, you just might make it. Don't let there be the slightest lull in conversation! Stall them with questions, like "I heard there was a new documentary about World War II submarine tactics—could you tell me more?" or "Have your neighbors done anything weird lately?" Or, alternatively, just start listing all the things that are going well in your life in the hope that it satisfies whatever parental angst they're having.

But the other option is to accept you're going to get wet and just let the downpour of conversation happen.

This is, frankly, what is probably going to happen anyway—even if you run, even if you redirect, even if you somehow make it through this particular visit without having a Big Conversation, it's going to happen sooner or later.

Sure, this deluge may leave you drenched and shivering. It may cause a lingering cold. And it may soak your shoes and make every movement heavier for a while. Or it might look like a storm but turn out to be just a sprinkle! You simply won't know the reality of their Big Conversation topic until you let the skies open up.

So let the rain come down, whatever winds and howls it brings. You're not going to melt, and having a Big Conversation isn't going to break you. Because after the storm passes, it will likely lead to clearer skies for the next visit. And if not? You'll know to bring an umbrella.

FOR WHEN YOU FORGOT TO REPLY TO THAT TEXT

A Template

Haven't replied to your friend's "Busy tonight?" text from three and a half months ago, and feeling like the biggest monster in the world about it?

Hey, it happens! Send them this handy dandy acronym that all the kids are using, they'll totally get it:

WIMSSIMSL8R2UPDTIPICWMTWIJTSLG2BSM&TAO C1AOMP(WIAHIMH)2OUTTUSM(WICSEWA2MIME WH)JSOS?TTIPCBGR8!I<3TNA2B&2TPLSOCWPB WTCAE&ATFIWIWJSHSTTA2S2AWEMOMP@AHOT DIDKMTNSGR84OLPB?TIA2SEF2ATSSGOBBL8TN SIMRNI<3UIRU&LNSOTA(UTNT1OUF2R)AWU2TW?

Which obviously means:

Wow, I am so sorry I'm so late replying to you! Please don't take it personally—it certainly wasn't meant that way. It's just that sometimes life gets to be so much, and the act of closing one app on my phone (which I already had in my hands) to open up the text you sent me (which,

I cannot stress enough, was available to me in my every waking hour) just seemed . . . overwhelming, somehow?

The thing is, phones can be great! I love the nonstop access to Bejeweled and to the "Personal Life" sections of celebrities' Wikipedia pages! But with that comes an ease and accessibility that, frankly, I wonder if we just shouldn't have. Suddenly, there's the ability to speak to anyone we've ever met on multiple platforms at all hours of the day. I don't know, maybe that's not so great for our little primate brains?

This is all to say: everyone forgets to answer texts sometimes. Shit gets overwhelming. But better late than never, so I'm replying now. I love you, I respect you, and let's never speak of this again (until the next time one of us forgets to reply). Anyway. Whatcha up to this weekend?

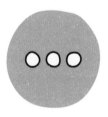

FOR WHEN YOU'RE THROWING A PARTY AND NO ONE'S HERE YET

Your guests are coming, we promise.

Just because you said "Come over at 7ish!" in the evite and it's currently 7:22 does not mean your guests all collectively decided to bail. They didn't seek out a rival party thrown by a slightly more fun friend who lives in a slightly more convenient neighborhood with a slightly more comprehensive party theme. You're great, your place is great, and your Golden Age of Cinema Murder Mystery Night is both fun and so historically accurate it could be peer-reviewed.

Maybe they're all just trying to be fashionably late to impress you and the other (very cool) attendees. Maybe they're all together at the store right now, buying you an impossibly extravagant hosting gift. Or maybe everyone accidentally spent twenty minutes staring at their phone in the bathroom when they should have been getting ready and are just now leaving the house. (Which is almost definitely what happened.)

So, before they all inevitably show up at the exact same time (except for that one friend who's always an hour-plus late to everything), take this time just for you.

Refill the bowl of Cool Ranch Doritos to replace the ones you just stress-ate. Practice your transatlantic accent one more time (not that you need to, it's perfect, dah-ling.) And enjoy the quiet before the laughter and murder accusations start flying.

Your guests are coming, we promise.

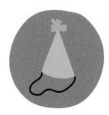

YOU

&

WORK

Personally, we think you're way too devilishly good-looking to have to work for a living. But until you win the lottery (try numbers 15-18-20-25-27, they just FEEL like winners!), here's some pep talks to get you through the day.

FOR WHEN YOU NEED TO GET THAT BORING WORK THING DONE

Honestly, if that one coworker has the confidence and the perseverance to show up late and leave early every day, then you can *definitely* work up the energy to get that one lingering item on your to-do list done.

Still not convinced? Here are ten other way less fulfilling things that will absolutely take the same amount of time and effort as just doing that boring work thing.

1. Considering taking (but not actually taking) a walk

2. Trying to remember what a Punnett square is

3. Thoroughly explaining the plot of a movie you saw once to a disinterested coworker

4. Attempting to figure out where your passport is (and when it expires)

5. Reading a recipe you'll never make

6. Googling your most forgettable middle school crush

7. Cleaning out the pockets of your least-used coat

8. Thinking about unsubscribing from all those marketing emails

9. Scrolling eBay to start your new Pez dispenser collection

10. Doing a different, unrelated work thing you've been putting off

FOR WHEN IT'S TIME FOR YOUR ANNUAL PERFORMANCE REVIEW

A Fill-in-the-Blank

Look, you're gonna crush your annual performance review. You're the freakin' best. In fact, your boss sent us an advance copy of your review and it's glowing—you just have to fill in a few details.

___[YOUR NAME]___, before we dive in, can I just say two words: *holy* ___[SWEAR WORD]___!!!! Apologies for my language, but frankly there's no other way to sum up your performance this year!!!!

Your work this year at ___[COMPANY YOU WORK AT]___ has been nothing short of ___[ADJECTIVE]___. Everything you touched—from ___[PROJECT YOU WORKED ON]___ to ___[ANOTHER PROJECT YOU WORKED ON]___—was worth more than a thousand ___[PLURAL EXPENSIVE OBJECT]___.

And your ___[THING YOU DO EVERY DAY]___ skills? I mean, that blew my ___[BODY PART]___ away. You alone earned this company more than ___[A LARGE NUMBER]___ buckaroos!

But ___[YOUR NAME]___—it's not just your skills and business prowess that makes you such a ___[ADJECTIVE]___ team player. It's also your ___[NICE TRAIT YOU HAVE]___. You make this place feel like more than a workplace—you make it feel like a ___[PLACE YOU LOVE TO SPEND TIME]___.

___[NICKNAME YOU'D LIKE TO HAVE]___—can I call you that? I just want to take a moment to say: You're more than just a ___[YOUR JOB TITLE]___ to me. You're like a ___[FAMILY MEMBER]___. Except even better, because I get to give you money . . . and this year, I'm giving you ___[EXORBITANTLY HIGH NUMBER]___ dollars.

You're the ___[SUPERLATIVE]___.

Sincerely,

___[YOUR BOSS'S NAME]___

FOR WHEN YOU HAVE TO SEND A SCARY EMAIL

A Foolproof Checklist

You can't just hover your mouse over SEND for forever. Plus, if you were to die under mysterious circumstances before you hit SEND and came back as a ghost, wouldn't you be *so* disappointed that sending this email was your unfinished business? You're too cool for that!

Follow this handy checklist, and you'll be sending that scary email out into cyberspace in no time.

☐ Did you spell the name(s) of the recipient(s) correctly?

☐ Did you confirm that you didn't accidentally call anyone "sweetie" or "shithead" or include the phrase "I love you" anywhere in the email?

☐ Did! You! Remove! Every! Unnecessary! Exclamation! Point?!?!?!?!

☐ Wait, is the email too cold now? Maybe add back in a couple of those exclamation points so you seem more likable!

☐ Read the email aloud to yourself. Be honest: does it sound like you, a Real Human Being, or more like you're an alien doing an impression of a Very Fancy Businessperson?

☐ Check again: Are you sure the names are right? Or did you put an *i* or *y* in the wrong place in Hayleigh?

☐ Is there anything in this email that you don't actually want to put in writing, for fear of it coming back to bite you later? Like your real thoughts about your boss or all your bank account information along with a comprehensive list of your passwords?

☐ Is any part of the email written in a font you'd describe as fun? (It's not. Remove it immediately.)

☐ If you said you attached a file, did you actually attach a file? And is it the correct file, or did you attach a top-secret file containing state secrets that an enemy planted on your computer to destabilize the government?

☐ Just check one more time—are you *sure* the name is right? If so, you're good to send!

FOR WHEN YOU SENT THE WRONG NAME IN AN EMAIL

A Foolproof Checklist

So you called somebody the wrong name in an email? It's okay, buddy! No matter how many checklists you have, things still fall through the cracks. It's not your fault. These things happen!

Now follow this checklist (but, like, actually follow it this time) to correct your mistake.

☐ Immediately draft an apology email. Please—and we cannot stress this enough—**check that you have the right name this time.**

☐ Send the email!

☐ Take a walk and think about what you've done. (Kidding! Go buy a little treat and remind yourself that you're doing your goddamn best and that's all you can do!)

FOR WHEN YOU'RE ASKING FOR A RAISE

Let's get down to business: this request for a raise needs to happen by EOD.

We don't need to boil the ocean on this one. You're clearly good at what you do. You're a collaborative teammate. You consistently hit your KPIs, your OKRs, your SMART goals, your CFOs, your ABCs, and your YMCAs. This company would be positively screwed without you.

And what's the worst that's going to happen? They say no? Well, let us save you a few thousand bucks on business school and tell you this: you've got to take all the shots you can, and that means missing sometimes, something, something, Michael Jordan, Wayne Gretzky, Ina Garten, et cetera. Whatever, you get it.

Career hack: it's never bad to remind your boss of all the reasons why you're deserving of a raise. When the rubber hits the road, there's only one person who's going to advocate for you at work—and that's you.

(And if we can just circle back for a quick sec: you're not asking for enough money. Ask for more. You're worth it!)

We've got a hard stop in fifty words, so here's the memo version: You've got moxie, kid. We know it, and they know it. Now go get that raise.

FOR WHEN THE CUSTOMER'S WRONG

Whoever said "the customer's always right" has definitely never met most customers. And today's customer is exploring new frontiers of just how wrong a customer can be. Like, so blatantly wrong that you feel insane even pointing it out.

Unfortunately, there's no pithy turn of phrase or devastatingly incisive comment that will make them say, "Gee, I was so wrong. Thank you for changing my life for the better, friend. Your constructive criticism has really inspired me!" You're stuck in the real-life version of an internet comments section: everyone's fired up, no one's ever going to agree, and the only way this ends is with you signing off.

So even though you're screaming on the inside, on the outside you're going to be as cool as a county-fair-blue-ribbon-winning cucumber. The Eagles once sang "You can't hide your lyin' eyes," but they were wrong (and also on a *lot* of drugs). In this case, lie away. Tell the customer you're "happy to help" or you'd be "glad to escalate this to management" or any other calm-sounding sentence that doesn't actually mean anything. The best way to defuse a bully is to deny them the fight they want (even if you really, really, *really* want to dress them down).

So while they may never hear the devastating retorts you'll rehearse in the shower later, you, without a doubt, would have absolutely decimated them with your intelligence and wit and commitment to the truth. And know that the next time they dare to step out of line, you'll be ready.

FOR WHEN YOU KNOW THAT ONE COWORKER WANTS TO CHIT-CHAT

The Board Game

David versus Goliath. The tortoise versus the hare. Predator versus the people in the movie that Predator fought. These stories are nothing compared to the showdown of the century: Our Brilliant Reader versus That One Coworker Who Just Wants to Chit-Chat.

Think you have what it takes to make it past That One Coworker without being pulled into a conversation about birds they've seen or a trip they took back in 2011? Or will you be stuck staying late to catch up on all the work you're behind on because you were trying to be polite?? If anyone can do it, it's you!

Let the game begin.

GAMEPLAY

1. Uh-oh! Looks like you need to pass That One Coworker's desk. Remember to bring your phone to intensely stare at as you walk past—if you make eye contact, go back to the beginning (and lose forty-five minutes out of your goddamn day).

2. Shoot! You're enjoying a leisurely lunch in the break room, shoving down a sandwich and staring at the wall when That One Coworker enters. Quick! Fake a sudden meeting that you "totally forgot about" or risk missing a deadline because they explained the entire plot to *Total Recall 2070: The TV Show* to you.

3. Phew! You've almost finished the game—but wait! As you're leaving for the day, That One Coworker is leaving at the same time—and boy, oh boy, do they have some thoughts on their new Hyundai Sonata. This is a toughie! If you've got kids, a pet, or a particularly finicky houseplant, throw them under the bus and say you need to rush home to them. If not, it looks like you lost this round—start again at the beginning tomorrow.

HOW TO WIN

You can't, really! Ultimately, you're gonna play this game every workday until you leave the company or until the other person loses their voice.

The thing is, That One Coworker wants to talk to you because you're a likable, interesting person who happens to also be within earshot. That's a compliment! But that also doesn't mean that you have to be their BFF—it's totally okay to talk to them when you have time and to put on your headphones and politely ignore them when you don't. That doesn't make you a bad person, that just makes you a person who has hit their limit on small talk.

Game on.

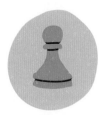

FOR WHEN EVERYONE AT WORK APPARENTLY TOOK STUPID PILLS TODAY

There are some days when work is easy. And then there's days like today, when everyone else apparently took stupid pills. By process of elimination, that makes you the smartest person here! Congrats!

That means today is basically a free pass for you. Totally beefed the big deadline? Robin didn't even know there *was* a deadline! Need to ask a question you've already asked eight times before? No one's going to care because Taylor just took down the entire server by enthusiastically replying to a spam email. Forgot the new guy's name? It's fine, Kelly just repeatedly called a client "Mom." No matter what you do, you're going to look like a total rock star (or at least like a decent second-tier rhythm guitarist) in comparison to all these fools.

And if you're feeling the pressure of holding the office together as the only sane, rational person today, stop. Unless you're a heart surgeon or the person in charge of making the ball drop on New Year's Eve, the whole world isn't going to come crashing down because everyone at work had an off day. All you have to worry about today is making it to quitting time.

FOR WHEN YOU WANT TO RAGE QUIT

An Interactive Saga

ONWARD, VALIANT WARRIOR! Now is your time to (metaphorically) burn this company to ash.

For too long have you endured the inane requests of your manager, and your so-called coworkers seem not to do any work. They are all weak and piteous—they grow lazy as they stuff their bellies with small talk and spreadsheets.

The only answer is (metaphorical) fire and (metaphorical) blood, and you will take what you are owed with the (allegorical) power of Thor's hammer. The spoils of the break room shall be yours!

Your time is now, and we will follow you into (corporate) battle wherever you lead!

DO YOU:

- Actually want to go through with it and rage quit? *If so, go to Path A.*

- Know you can't rage quit, but want to make a little trouble? *If so, go to Path B.*

- Mostly feel better now, if you're being honest with yourself? *If so, go to Path C.*

Path A

Hoist your mighty resignation letter and strike true on the desk of your manager. When you are done here, all that shall remain is a trail of scorched receipts for reimbursement and the shattered egos of those who have wronged you. Ride forth and take your place in the halls of Valhalla, mighty warrior!

Path B

Though you chose peace today, this indignity cannot go unchecked. Take thou a long lunch and avail thyself of mead (or Diet Coke), warrior! Take a sick day when thou art not sick! Start a little rumor about Karl from Accounting—nothing horrible, but enough to make people whisper!

Path C

Only the wisest of warriors know when to swing their sword and when to show mercy. Bide your time—these lowly peasants disgust you, but they can prove useful in the long run, maybe for a reference or an intro via LinkedIn. Turn your sights to the horizon, for there are other, more bountiful companies to explore.

FOR WHEN YOU FEEL LIKE YOU'RE ABOUT TO GET FIRED

There are only two types of workdays: the days when you think that your workplace would collapse into a zillion pieces without you there, and the days when it feels like you're one false step away from being canned.

And buddy, today you're having one of the latter.

Regardless of what (if anything!) you did, the reality is it's a lot of work to fire someone. The awkward conversations! The meetings with HR! The comically large mountain of paperwork! Firing someone is truly a pain in the butt, especially when that someone is as smart and capable and charismatic as you.

There could be a million reasons for the workplace vibes feeling off today, from Bill leaving stale donuts in the break room (dammit, Bill), to everyone else simply running around worried that *they're* about to get fired. The possibilities are endless!

So, while there's really no way for us to know for sure (your boss didn't reply to our numerous meeting invites to circle back on this), we're pretty sure you're not going to get fired today.

FOR WHEN YOU ACTUALLY ARE FIRED

First off, we really beefed that one. As it turns out, there are actually *three* types of workdays: the ones when it feels like that place can't function without you, the ones when you feel like you're about to be fired, and the rare ones when you actually *are* fired. And it looks like you're having that last one.

That sucks. A lot. It probably feels unlucky, unfair, and deeply unwarranted. (Unless you did something wild like upload all the files on your work computer to an online forum called "STEAL FROM MY COMPANY LOL," in which case . . . maybe you need a different type of pep talk from a different type of book.)

You're going to get through this. This shitty event will one day be nothing more than a line on your resume—a resume that, with an all-star brain (and an all-star boo-ty) like yours, we're sure will also feature job titles like "President of Earth" and "CFO of Big Business" (or, you know, the equivalent titles for whatever industry you're in).

So do what you need to do to get through the next few days. Go on a walk during business hours. Buy yourself a little "I've been fired" treat. Write a scathing review of your boss, then throw it in the toilet. And then put yourself back out there.

FOR WHEN YOU'VE ALREADY ASKED WHAT EVERYONE AT LUNCH DID LAST WEEKEND AND NOW YOU'RE OUT OF THINGS TO TALK ABOUT

Well, shoot. You've been sitting silently in the break room for five full minutes, listening to Dan eat his (weirdly wet) salad, and there's no sign of someone else restarting the conversation. It looks like saving this work lunch has somehow fallen squarely onto your shoulders. You didn't wake up today and decide to be a hero—and yet here you are.

You got this. You're the Dolly Parton of this office—folksy, iconic, and capable of writing multiple number one hit songs in a day. But if you're drawing a blank, here are a few suggestions to kickstart this lunch back to life.

- The weather (current, past, upcoming, in general, in comparison to elsewhere, etc.)

- The office chairs: do we like them?

- Computers: pretty wild, right? If you really think about it!

- Weird nicknames everyone has for their pets (and we need pictures)

- Concerts (specific ones)

- Concerts (in general)

- Your 1997–1998 Chicago Bulls!!!!!!!

- Water: is everyone drinking enough of it?

- Take bets on how many sick days Chuck has used so far this year

- Is it just you or has the printer been acting weird this week?

- Who's seen a ghost?

- What do you think happens after you die?

- Politics! (Just kidding.)

- How many states can you name?

- What's everyone's salary?!? (Who deserves more? Who deserves *less*?)

- Who's gotten scammed before?

- What's everyone eating? How appetizing does it look to you, personally?

- Has everyone seen a bat before? (Some people haven't!)

- Has everyone done their HR training?

- What everyone's going to do *next* weekend?

Remember: it's not what you say, but how you say it. And with your natural charisma and Oscar-worthy delivery, any one of these topics is going to get the lunch table talking.

FOR WHEN YOU'RE OUT OF VACATION DAYS

First off, here's hoping that you used up all your vacation days on something really fun, like solving a mystery aboard a transatlantic cruise or competing in—and ultimately winning—*Survivor: All-Stars*. But whatever the reason, here you are: fresh out of vacation days and hankering for your next adventure (or at least a day away from your coworkers).

Look, this sucks. If it was up to us, you'd have a cushy six-figure job as the nation's premier luxury resort tester. But ultimately, vacation is all about giving yourself experiences outside of your ordinary routine. And, sure, that's ideally done while sipping a frozen marg on the sands of CocoCay, the official private island of Royal Caribbean cruises, but you don't need your boss's approval to make the most of your nonworking hours.

Instead, set plans that make the everyday feel special. Get an overpriced seasonal latte from a new coffee shop during your break! Visit a tourist attraction in your own town that you've never actually been to! (Bonus points if your hometown happens to have the World's Largest Ball of Twine.) Convince your boss to change all the clocks to "island time," whatever the heck that means!

And if all else fails, there's always sick days.

YOU
&
ROMANCE

Love is patient, love is kind . . .
and sometimes love is also a huge pain
in the ass. Wherever you are in your
romantic endeavors, we're there too.
(Metaphorically speaking, of course.)

FOR WHEN YOU HAVE A LITTLE CRUSH

A News Alert

PLANET EARTH—Reader has a little crush on someone, a panel of experts announced at a news conference today.

The astonishing proclamation sent shockwaves through members of the press, amazed onlookers, and longtime big ol' fans of Reader, who gathered to hear the report.

"The rumors are true," said Dr. Jericah P. Smoochworthy, Professor of Infatuation Studies at the University of K-I-S-S-I-N-G. "I'm thrilled to announce today that Reader has a little crush. It's an update that is completely understandable because, as we often say in the academic community, the world is filled with so many grade-A hotties, crushes are bound to happen."

Dr. Smoochworthy reassured attendees that Reader doesn't have to blow up their whole life just because they have a little crush on someone, and that they're welcome to ride out this fun little distraction while it lasts. (However, ten out of ten experts agree that Crush is probably into Reader too, because how could they not be?)

"Whether Reader wants to make a move or simply wants to sit back and enjoy the fun of a crush—such as bouts of daydreaming and excuses to wear their 'good shirt'—we experts are in unanimous agreement: this is fun and not bad," Dr. Smoochworthy said.

Dr. Smoochworthy also noted that, statistically speaking, there's almost definitely people out there who, in turn, have a crush on Reader, whether or not Reader knows it.

"And how could they not?" Dr. Smoochworthy demanded of the audience. "Reader is smart, talented, and cool as hell. You'd be a fool not to have a crush on them."

More updates are expected later this week.

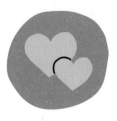

CORRECTION: An earlier version of this article egregiously omitted that Reader was also smart and talented, on top of being "cool as hell." The article has been updated to reflect reality.

FOR WHEN YOU'RE GETTING BACK ON THE DATING APPS (AGAIN)

Well, it finally happened. You downloaded those stupid little dating apps (again).

Let's face it. Nobody really wants to be back on the dating apps (again), still using that profile picture from Coachella three years ago that we all know needs to be swapped out for something more recent.

But redownloading the apps is actually an act of bravery. It's brave to be vulnerable, it's brave to take steps toward finding happiness and, heck, it's even brave to fib about your height by two to four inches or so. Remember—you are on the apps, the apps aren't on you. (Okay, that doesn't actually mean anything. But doesn't it sound inspirational?)

So while you wait for that "Forgot password?" email to come through, remember the three cardinal rules of dating on the apps that you're gonna stick to this time.

1. **You're going to have a personality.** You are a vibrant, interesting, attractive, funny person. So why does your profile say something as generic as "I love travel!"? Of course you do! Everyone loves travel! That's why flights cost $5,000!

There's no need to airbrush your profile until anyone else's name could be on it. Maybe you really *are* a six-foot-tall fisherman who loves "hanging out" and "the weekend." But maybe you're *actually* the owner of the world's largest troll doll collection—which is *way* more interesting and, frankly, will help your troll-loving soulmate find you even faster!

2. **You're going to be intentional.** You came here for a reason. If that reason is to find a long-term companion or to try new experiences, go ahead and be up front about it. And if you're simply looking to touch as many people's butts as humanly possible in the next thirty days, then make that clear from the get-go (and we hope you touch a minimum of sixty consenting cheeks).

3. **You're going to lower your expectations.** Look, we've all heard about that friend of a friend who married the first person they matched with. But much like Bigfoot and an electable third-party presidential candidate, that is just an urban legend and not an expectation you should plan your life around. If you meet the right person on the apps, that's great! But if all you have are a couple of flirty conversations and mediocre dates, then that's okay, too. You're putting yourself out there, and that's what matters.

So take a deep breath and get back to swiping (again). We think you'll surprise yourself, and you'll be a welcome surprise to others.

FOR WHEN YOU'RE ABOUT TO SEE YOUR EX

Ideally, post-breakup, all exes would be sent to a farm upstate, where they could spend their days roaming free, sending passive-aggressive texts, and not committing to anyone or anything. But until the bank finally gives us a small business loan to break ground on Old MacDonald's Fuckup Farm, you're going to be stuck occasionally seeing your ex.

Despite what it may feel like, you don't have to prove anything to your former paramour. No matter how it feels in this moment, you're a smart, attractive, lovable person. Don't stress about showing them that you "won" the breakup. (Even though we all know that you totally wiped the floor with them.)

Whether this meetup feels just like old times or you throw a drink right in their dumb face (please, please, try your best not to do that)—you can get through this. Just like your relationship with them, this interaction won't last forever.

FOR WHEN YOU JUST GOT GHOSTED

A Spooky Tale

A raven screeches, the wind howls through the trees, and a jack-o-lantern sits sort of ominously on a stoop

One dark and stormy night, an earnest, kindhearted individual put themselves out there and took a brave step into the dark, unforgiving forest that is the modern dating scene.

They swiped, they messaged, they grabbed drinks, they asked strangers inane questions about siblings and TV shows. And no matter how unhinged their dates' answers were, our kindhearted hero pretended to actually care.

And then, after repeating this process for many a full moon, our hero finally thought they found a good match.

Until one night, that good match . . . disappeared without a trace.

The kindhearted individual searched high and low for them—they looked at their social media profiles, they asked mutual friends, they even sent a few "Hey, how's your week?" text messages to the missing person.

But no matter what they did, they heard only a deathly silence. It was as if this supposedly good match had simply . . . vanished.

OOOO₀₀₀₀₀₀₀OOOOOOO₀₀₀₀₀₀₀₀₀₀₀₀₀OOO*ohhhh*

Shhhhh. Did you hear that?! It couldn't be . . .

Sound of chains rattling

Oh no! It's the most horrifying thing of all: the gh-gh-gh-ghostly presence of an emotionally immature person on the dating scene! AHHHHHH!!!

But wait! While a ghosting seems impossibly scary, it's actually a *lot* less terrifying than the alternative: wasting any more time with someone who doesn't realize just how special you are.

That doesn't make being stood up hurt any less. But this ghost of a date isn't your unfinished business to carry around, to obsess over and regret. In fact, this isn't on you at all—it's on them. (And that's a problem for them and their ghost therapist to figure out.)

So do what you would do for any haunting: perform some kind of banishing ritual, swap spooky stories about this ghost with your friends and, when you're ready, re-lease the thought of them back into the ether.

You go, ghoul.

FOR WHEN YOU WANT TO ASK SOMEONE OUT ON A DATE

A Top-Secret Mission

OPERATION: MEET-CUTE
TOP-SECRET MISSION. HIGH PRIORITY.
CARRY OUT IMMEDIATELY.

Your mission, should you choose to accept it, is to ask the target CODENAME: CRUSH out on a date.

No one else has the right mix of good looks, spunk, and all-around appeal to pull this off—it has to be you.

Be on alert for the right time to intercept CODENAME: CRUSH and ask them out on a date. Do not miss your window; there may not be another opportunity.

All our intelligence suggests the following:

1. You're a catch, and CODENAME: CRUSH would be lucky to go on a date with you.

2. You deserve to put yourself out there.

3. The vibes are real.

Stick to your emotional counterintelligence training—keep it clean and simple. Get in, make the request, and get out. No fluffy stuff like "I was wondering if you maybe, sometime, might be interested in possibly . . ." Direct, declarative sentences like "Hey, I like talking with you, would you like to go out sometime?" Once you get the answer, get out of there before your mouth stops working and you say something dumb like "Catch you on the flip side, crocodile."

Good luck, we're all counting on you.

OPERATIONAL ALERT

If CODENAME: CRUSH is at their place of work, abort operation immediately.

UPON COMPLETION OF MISSION

Text a friend to let them know how it went.

DESTROY THIS DOCUMENT* AFTER READING

Catch you on the flip side, crocodile,
Your handler

---

* Go to the next page, please don't destroy this book, we worked so hard on it!!!

FOR WHEN YOUR CRUSH STARTS DATING SOMEONE ELSE

If you were an Olive Garden entrée, everyone knows you'd be the crown jewel: Lasagna Classico.

But even if you're the cheesiest, gooiest, most simultaneously saucy-but-flaky, most amazing Lasagna Classico in the world (and you are), there's still gonna be some people out there who order the Never-Ending Soup and Salad instead.

That doesn't mean there's anything wrong with lasagna! (Remember: you're the lasagna.) Lasagna is still a fan favorite! The Tour of Italy platter would be nothing without you! You're front and center on the menu for a reason!

Still, that doesn't mean that lasagna is going to be every person's preference. How devastatingly boring would that be? Menus listing nothing but lasagna? Streets lined with lasagna-only restaurants? Saturday morning cartoon commercials filled with lasagna-based cereals, like Capitano Crunch's "Mama Mia! All Lasagna!"? It'd be overwhelming for you, and devastating for everyone who's gluten free. (Bear with us. You're still the lasagna here somehow.)

Although it feels frustrating and sad that people are ordering basic, boring unlimited soup and salad when what you're offering is so wonderful, there's someone out there who is dreaming of finding exactly the kind of lasagna you are. They're telling their friends about the lasagna they're searching for, they're imagining what life with the lasagna will be like, they're downloading apps to find the perfect lasagna for them. (Once again, you're the lasagna, and they're downloading a hybrid Olive Garden rewards/delivery/dating app. Don't think too hard about it.)

Luckily, you're now unencumbered by that soup and salad eater, so go out there and find the lasagna lover of your dreams.

We believe in you. Because when you're here, you're family.

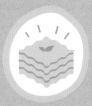

FOR WHEN EVERYONE SEEMS TO BE IN A RELATIONSHIP BUT YOU

Yet another Saturday night of going out in your least wrinkled shirt, paying for your own cocktails, and revising your dating profiles in the bar bathroom? You're not alone (though it sure may feel like it right now).

But, much like ancient sailors who were lured to the rocks by a siren's song, only to be crushed to death by a pissed-off walrus, being in a relationship isn't always the mythical promised land that it's cracked up to be. Just because everyone else is jumping overboard doesn't mean you have to settle for the next singing marine mammal you come across.

In this moment, you might be wondering if you made the right call to stay single and not shack up. The answer is yes! Sure, being in a relationship has its benefits, but it also means constantly meeting halfway. How exhausting! You have to consider someone else's bedtime, dietary restrictions, and (God forbid) questionable taste in movies and TV. And then there's the big stuff, like communicating emotions and always having to do couples Halloween costumes. (Sometimes you want to dress up as just *one* of the Ghostbusters!)

Meanwhile, being single is great! You get to do whatever you want, whenever you want. No gods, no masters!

Pee with the door open! Flirt with everyone! Pull an *Under the Tuscan Sun* by flying to Italy, buying an abandoned villa, and filling your closet with crisp linen shirts! Anything is possible!

Part of the fun of this single era is not knowing what the future holds. You're steering your own boat, and you're free to stop at whatever port makes you happy. If you find a spot to drop anchor—great! And if you're having fun cruising the open seas, that's great, too!

Fair winds and following seas, solo sailor!

FOR WHEN EVERYONE SEEMS TO BE SINGLE BUT YOU

Yet another Saturday night of staying in with your partner, wearing *mostly* clean sweatpants, drinking a beer that's been in the fridge since your housewarming party, and scrolling through post after post of your single friends living it up? Your relationship is great, but it's hard to not feel like you're missing out right now.

There's a reason that none of the good rom-coms have sequels. There's no *You've Got Mail at Your Joint Address* or *When Harry Went Splitsies with Sally on a New Lawnmower*. That's because after the exciting start, a good relationship naturally gets a little boring. There's no tense "will they or won't they" moments or dramatic proclamations of love at the airport after you've helped them pick out a sleep apnea machine.

In this moment, you might be wondering if you made the right call to hitch your wagon to this (loudly snoring) person. The answer is yes! Sure, being single has its benefits, but it also means a lot of surface-level connections and alone time. How exhausting! You're constantly staying up late, you have to do all the chores by yourself, and if you want to go on dates again (God forbid), they're mainly stinkers! And then there's the big stuff, like existential dread and coming up with a hot but funny Halloween costume. (Will people get your sexy Egon Spengler outfit?)

Meanwhile, being in a relationship is great! You get to hang out with your best friend all the time! It's you two against the world! Have a chat in the bathroom while one of you pees! Unapologetically reference your own inside jokes! Pull a *Mr. and Mrs. Smith* by dressing nicely, having fulfilling careers, and joining forces to take down the shadow organizations that employ you both! Anything is possible!

Part of the fun of this partnered era is not knowing what the future holds but getting to go forward into it together. While you may not have a need to stand outside your partner's window holding a boom box, that's only because you already share a Spotify account and because you can only take so many minutes of their "Groovy Weekday Morning" playlist.

So roll the credits and enjoy your (occasionally boring) Hollywood ending.

FOR WHEN YOU WANT TO SAY "I LOVE YOU" FOR THE FIRST TIME

Break out the heart-shaped confetti! Sprinkle rose petals on whatever surfaces are in sight! Blast Brian McKnight's greatest hits! You're ready to say you're in love! How exciting is this?!?

Yes, it might be physically painful and emotionally draining and intellectually distracting, but we are thrilled you have found someone you feel so strongly about. We promise this is the good kind of nausea!

Telling someone you love them doesn't have to be particularly smooth or planned out. All it has to be is genuine. If it helps you to write it in a note, then go off, Shakespeare! If you and your lover enjoy theatrical displays of affection, then hire two planes to kiss in the sky! And if the words spontaneously fall out of your face and you kind of yell them in the process, then that's perfect, too!

We know what you're thinking: what happens if they don't say it back? No matter what happens, you're doing an incredibly brave and vulnerable thing. At least you'll know where you stand! What a relief! That sure beats an unsaid "I love you" eating you from the inside out like a ravenous parasite. Plus, you're a total catch—if they don't feel the same way, that sounds like a them problem!

No matter what happens, you've got this. (Love you.)

FOR WHEN YOU'RE INTRODUCING A NEW PARTNER TO YOUR FRIENDS

As five wise British women once said, "If you wanna be my lover, you gotta get with my friends." Well, Monogamy Spice, it's your turn to step into the spotlight, because your new partner is about to meet *your* friends.

We'll tell you what we want (what we really, really want): for you to not freak out about this.

Don't get us wrong, this is a big deal. Whether this is the first partner your friends have ever met or simply the latest person to Spice Up Your Life, making this introduction is always a major milestone.

But this is a good thing, not a Scary one! It's a natural, necessary next step if you truly want 2 Become 1. Plus, what's the alternative? Your partner never meeting your friends? Oh, pish Posh! You like this person, and you want them to be a larger part of your life!

Here's the secret, Baby: the more confidently you introduce your partner, the more excited everyone will be. There's no reason to treat it Gingerly. This is the time to trust it, use it, prove it, groove it, show how good you are together!

No matter how the intro goes, remember that

friendship never ends. If today goes well, then that's great! If it *doesn't* go well, there will be more chances! Your friends want you to be happy, and if you're really excited about this new partner, they'll be a good Sporty about getting to know them.

(Zigazig, ah.)

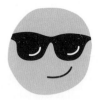

FOR WHEN YOUR PARTNER'S JUST KIND OF BEING ANNOYING

There's a million little reasons why you love your partner. The adorable way they hold their coffee cup. The focused face they make when they're thinking. The gentle way they readjust their glasses.

But today, everything about them is annoying as hell. The stupid way they hold their coffee cup. The stupid face they make when they're thinking. The especially stupid way they can't stop readjusting their stupid glasses.

We're here to tell you that your feelings are valid. Even if everything else is exactly the same, sometimes the energy's just off. Just because you love your partner doesn't mean you have to always like them. Nothing's all good 100 percent of the time, not even Bruce Springsteen songs. (Sometimes it just needs more saxophone, Boss!)

So change it up. Go take a walk! Move to a different room (or side of the room if space is tight)! Put on your headphones and stare at a screen for a while! (Especially if it's to watch a show that you love and they "just don't get.")

We promise this will pass, and your partner will go back to being the object of your affection. But until then? Get some distance between yourself and four-eyes.

FOR WHEN YOU GET DUMPED

Against all odds, you—a radiant, kind, intelligent gift from the universe—have been dumped. There's no way to sugarcoat it: it sucks, it's bad, and frankly, it's shocking!

If there were a series of words that would magically fix that ache in the pit of your stomach, please know that we would write them in a heartbeat. Wait, let's just try it: Aquifer. Labradoodle. Caravan. Monopoly Man. Did that work? Did we fix it? Are you feeling better yet?!?

Ultimately, with heartbreaks—much like the Lincoln Tunnel and the 2022 film *Morbius*—the only way out is through. There's a certain kind of freedom that comes with being dumped, a societal hall pass for deeply feeling your feelings and doing whatever the heck you want. So it's time to make like a mid-2000s #GirlBoss and #LeanIn. Consider this your invitation to wallow.

Don't know where to start? Well, lucky for you, we are the world's preeminent experts on the act of wallowing. And, kiddo, we're assigning you some homework. Do what makes you feel better, then repeat until you've forgotten your ex's birthday.

- **Buy yourself a cake.** One secret that Big Vegetable doesn't want you to know is that you don't need to wait for a birthday to buy a cake. The grocery store will sell you one on any day, for any reason. Eat it with your hands!

- **Silently lie on your bed.** Imagine you're the lead in a play about heartbreak. Consider the possibility that you've created the next great Broadway show. Furiously google "What to wear to Tony Awards?"

- **Think about getting bangs.** Resist all you want, but the siren song of bangs comes for us all. Do it or don't, there's nothing we can do to stop you.

- **Watch yourself cry in the mirror.** Start thinking about how beautiful you look when you cry. You're a model. A muse. Any artist would be lucky to paint you.

- **Make plans with your friends, then consider bailing, then decide to go anyway.** Stay out all night or come home crying after thirty minutes. Anything goes.

- **Put on a movie that you've seen no fewer than 350 times.** Restart it again the second it's over. Repeat until you no longer know where the movie ends and reality begins.

- **Remember that sometimes, it's cliché because it's true.** In this case, the phrase in question is "there are many other fish in the sea"—including ones that are going to see you for the incredible, joyful, amazing starfish you are.

YOU
&
THE BIG
STUFF

Need a pep talk with just a dash of
existential dread? Buddy, we've all
been there. We're in this together.

FOR WHEN IT'S MONDAY

An Op-Ed

Hey everyone, Monday here. And boy, oh boy, am I ever pissed off!!!

I bought space in this book to defend myself once and for all from the absolute onslaught of Monday slander out there. "A case of the Mondays"? "Blue Monday"?? "Monday Night Football"?!?! I mean, where do you people get off?!

Look, I'm not entirely blaming a certain orange comic strip cat for this defamation of my character, but I certainly don't think he did me any favors. But here's the thing: you'd never consider feeding your cat a full tray of lasagna every day, so why would you listen to him about Mondays sucking?

Much like street pigeons, cauliflower, and early 2000s television teen dramas (RIP, *One Tree Hill*), I have an undeserved bad rap. I've gone through a *lot* of therapy to learn to love myself. And now I'm here to set the record straight, once and for all.

I get it. I'll never be as carefree as Sunday Funday, as delicious as Taco Tuesday, or as irresponsible as Blackout Drunk Thursday. But I still have a lot of great qualities! I'm fresh-faced! I'm the start of something new! I'm a great excuse for an overpriced coffee! I'm a goddamn dream!

This week is starting whether you like it or not, and the possibilities are freaking endless. This week, you could get your dream job! You could check that one looming thing off your to-do list! You could finally achieve the perfectly timed commute! And it all starts with me, Good Ol' Reliable Monday.

Go get 'em, Nermal.

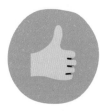

FOR WHEN YOU FREAK YOURSELF OUT THINKING ABOUT HOW BIG THE UNIVERSE IS

You didn't mean for it to happen. You were minding your own business, thinking about Jupiter's moons again (why are there so many?!), and then WHAM! Your brain blasted off on a terrifying tour of how big the universe is, how small we really are, and—because you're extra lucky today—how a mere several billion years from now, the sun is going to explode. And now you're fully freaked out.

It's going to be okay. Having a Semiannual Moment of Existential Panic™ is a natural side effect of being human! On the one hand, humans are so incredibly smart. We invented tools! We developed written language! There's been, like, a dozen versions of *Mario Kart*! On the other hand, this also means we can grasp human insignificance in the grand opera of space. It all comes with the territory.

It's equal parts unsettling and inspiring. And there's also nothing you—or anyone else—can do about it.

It's not like some of us are tiny specks on a rock floating through an ever-expanding universe and some of us aren't—every single person, plant, animal, and tchotchke that you've ever interacted with is in the same boat (or, more accurately, on the same planet). There's no changing any of it. However you want to slice it and whatever your beliefs are, we're all, ultimately, in this together.

So take a deep breath. Blink a few times. If needed, apologize to the other guests at this dinner party for screaming, "OH GOD, OH GOD!!" suddenly and without warning. And keep on living your best, deeply human life: blissfully unaware that you're not the center of the universe.

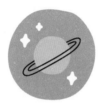

FOR WHEN YOU'RE LIVING SMACK-DAB IN ANXIETY CITY

A Real Estate Listing

Welcome to this stunning residence located in the heart of Anxiety City! Nestled right in between Why Did I Say That Dumb Thing Eight Years Ago? Avenue[1] and Is Everyone Mad at Me? Boulevard,[2] this is a rare opportunity to own property in the City That Never Sleeps Well.

Say hello to the open floor plan of your dreams, perfect for nervously pacing circles at 3 AM as you think about everything you've ever done and everything that could ever happen. (Oh là là!) And if you're a big entertainer, then you are going to *love* deciding to host a party and then nervously lying on this brand-new plush carpeting at 8:05 PM, wondering if anyone is actually going to show up![3] (Party monster alert!) And did we mention the breakfast nook?!

Whatever your goals are and however you most like to panic about the possibility of never achieving them, this little slice of hell in Anxiety City can be all yours for the low, low cost of a lifetime of heart palpitations, shortness

---

[1] See page 22.
[2] See page 92.
[3] See page 106.

of breath, and a constant knot in the pit of your stomach!

But wait—before you fork over that down payment, have you considered the fact that you don't actually have to *move* to Anxiety City?

It's true! Just because you're currently in town doesn't mean that you have to pick up all your baggage and fully take up residence. Billions of people visit Anxiety City every day. Whether you're in town for the afternoon because you drank one too many cups of coffee[4] or if you've been here for months on an extended vacation, this trip—like all other trips—will eventually end, no matter how it feels right now. And you'll be free to buy property in GoodVibesville, where you deserve to be.

[4] See page 36.

FOR WHEN THE NEWS IS TOO MUCH

The news can be an overwhelming, devastating cacophony of every fear you've ever had (and all the fears you didn't know even existed yet) muddled together in a terrifying, chunky stew. It's devastating earthquakes meets conspiracy theorists meets gruesome true crime meets *E. coli* in the romaine lettuce meets something called "Extra Buff Sewer Rats." And—at least in this moment—there's (probably) nothing you personally can do to single-handedly fix it.

And isn't that kind of freeing? No matter how passionate you are about the issues, this isn't on you alone to solve! World leaders aren't breathlessly ringing you up in the middle of the night to ask you to fix things for them, stat. (Unless you're a literal United Nations delegate, in which case ignore all of this! Fix things! Please! Hurry!!!!)

Constantly refreshing your phone to stay updated on every breaking news alert will just send you into an endless Wolf Blitzer–fueled spiral. You're not a vigilante tasked with monitoring all updates everywhere. You're a person with obligations, a social life, and (just a hunch here) at least a light to middling case of anxiety. Stepping away from the news doesn't make you uncaring or complicit—it makes you a human being whose brain isn't meant to constantly consume information on every global tragedy all at once. In order to do good in the world, you have to do good for yourself, too.

So take a moment to stop doomscrolling and find something that will make your day just 3 percent better. That doesn't have to be throwing your phone into the depths of the sea (both because that's expensive and also because, as you well know from all the news you've just consumed, the sea has enough problems already). Maybe it's taking a flattering picture of your pet. Maybe it's reminiscing about a great sandwich you ate once. Maybe it's still scrolling the news, but doing it outside.

And remember that even as breaking news unfolds in real time all around us, the world is still full of good people and everyday acts of kindness. The good always exists alongside the bad. Your newsfeed may be overwhelmingly full of devastating stories, but that doesn't mean that positive things aren't happening—it just means that they're so commonplace that they're not even worth reporting on. (Let's be honest here, "Two Old Friends Hug at Airport" is a pretty boring headline.) Focusing on small joys for a while is, we guarantee you, not going to make anything *worse*—and depriving yourself of those good things isn't going to reverse any earthquakes or decontaminate any lettuce.

This just in: you're a good person for caring about the world this much. But you gotta make sure you're caring about yourself, too.

FOR WHEN YOU'RE GRIEVING

Frequently True Clichés

Whatever you're grieving—whether it's the loss of a loved one, a dream that wasn't realized, or simply the end of an era—we are so sorry for your loss.

So much of what's said about grief can feel cliché. But while nothing will fully encapsulate the deeply personal experience you're going through, the thing about clichés is that they're often cliché for a reason. Sometimes they're played out, but sometimes they hold a universal truth that can serve as a path forward (or at least feel comforting at a time when comfort is hard to come by).

So here's a list of clichés about grief. Take in the ones that resonate today (or this hour or this minute) and ignore the others. Same goes for tomorrow and the day after that.

Frequently True Clichés About Grief

- Grief is grief. You're not dumb or weak for feeling it, regardless of the cause or timeline or size. And you are certainly not going to push it down to deal with later.

- Grief is exhausting! God, it's so exhausting, isn't it? Wouldn't it be nice to have the energy for literally anything else?? It'd be so much easier if grief made you sad *and* want to do the dishes!

- Grief is lonely. Regardless of your support system, it's deeply isolating to live so much inside your own feelings.

- Grief isn't about "should." There's no specific "way you should feel by now" or "things you should be doing to feel better." The only thing you *should* be doing is taking care of yourself, however you can.

- Grief is like a toddler. At any given moment, it might be messy, it might kick and punch you in the gut, and it might refuse to go to bed when all you want is to go to sleep. But sometimes, it might be filled with laughter, it might be inquisitive, and it might do something that stops you in your tracks with awe.

- Grief can make you feel like you're forgetting, and frankly that can feel like loss all over again. But you're not betraying anyone by forgetting small details, and it doesn't diminish the time you spent together.

- Grief is another form of love. You're hurting because you loved so big, and that kind of love stays with you forever.

- And one more frequently true cliché: you're going to be okay.

FOR WHEN YOU REALLY BEEFED IT, BIG TIME

WOOHOO! HELL YEAH! YOU BEEFED IT BIG TIME, BABY! ASSEMBLE THE BALLOON ARCH! PUT ON KOOL & THE GANG, AND LET'S CELEBRATE GOOD TIMES (C'MON)!

Maybe you beefed it in a very public way. Maybe you beefed it in an unnecessarily expensive way. Or maybe you just beefed it in a way that was so deeply embarrassing all you want to do is pack your bags and move into a faraway cave, where you can spend your days eating dirt sandwiches and befriending vermin and pretending that none of this ever happened.

However you beefed it, we're so freaking proud of you.

Beefing it big time is simply a sign that you're interesting. It's a sign that you're trying new shit out—shit that may not always work the way you wanted it to, but the point is that you're trying new shit in the first place. You're learning! You're growing! You're fucking up so spectacularly that you feel like you may have ruined your own life! How exciting is that?!

You know who doesn't ever beef it big time? Boring people. And that's because they're so scared of making massive mistakes that they end up just beefing their whole life away.

But that's not you.

You definitely beefed it this time—we're not denying that. But that's kind of what life is: beefing it again, and again, and again. You're gonna beef it in ways that you didn't even know was possible to beef something. You're gonna beef it so much and so often that you'll barely remember this specific instance of beefing it.

And every single one of those times should be celebrated.

Pick up the pieces as best you can. Delete the evidence. Hire a team of tight-lipped and incredibly thorough professional cleaners. And then get back out there and beef it some more.

FOR WHEN YOU'RE CELEBRATING A WIN (OF ANY SIZE)

Hey—congrats! You did it! Great work! Now go celebrate your win!

It doesn't matter how big (landing your dream job!) or small (the dentist complimented your commitment to flossing!), it's important to celebrate your successes.

Frankly, we were worried you might not celebrate yourself at all. So we got you a little something. We know, we know, we didn't have to, but we're just so proud of you!

CERTIFICATE OF UNDENIABLE SUCCESS

In recognition of the personal win(s) of

_____

[YOUR NAME]

_____

This certificate acknowledges that the above party absolutely, 100 percent,
totally crushed it. Truly a triumph of the highest order. A grand slam.
Way to go! You deserve a little treat (or twenty).

Paula Skaggs

CHANCELLOR OF CELEBRATION

Josh Linden

DEAN OF SUCCESS STUDIES

FOR WHEN SOMETHING IS ENDING

A Yearbook Sign-Off

Dear Reader,

So you've reached it. The end of the road. The final count-down. The last M&M in the bag of trail mix. Something you love is ending—whether it's a trip, an experience, a life chapter, or (just maybe) the last page in a book you (hopefully) loved.

Everything comes to an end, blah, blah, blah. You already know that, babycakes! But that doesn't make it any less bittersweet.

There's an infinite number of amazing things that are going to happen to you throughout your life—and wow, are those things going to rule!—but to get to those, some current adventures have to wrap up.

So close out this chapter in whatever way feels most right to you. Throw a rager, make an overly emotional photo slideshow, start a (controlled) cleansing fire—anything will do, just as long as it gives you a chance to properly say goodbye.

And remember what our good friends, the band Semisonic, once said: "Every new beginning comes from some other beginning's end." (We have never met Semisonic, but we do think we'd vibe.)

This summer is going to rule.

HAGS. LYLAS.
U R 2 SWEET
2 B 4GOTTEN.

—Paula and Josh

Gah! We tried as hard as we could, but it turned out to be nearly impossible to write a pep talk for every conceivable human experience within 176 pages. (If only we had 177!) So here's some DIY Tiny Pep Talks for you to customize, so you're prepared for whatever comes your way.

FOR WHEN _____

A DIY Tiny Pep Talk for When Something Bad Is Happening

Hey there, [CIRCLE ONE] BUDDY / TIGER / HONEY / YOU.

We're so sorry to hear about [BAD THING]. And when the going gets tough, even the toughest among us (like you, Tony Soprano, and Olympic figure skaters who just beefed the triple axel) need a little pep talk. So here goes.

There's no way around it: going through [BAD THING] is absolutely [CIRCLE ONE] STRESSFUL / ANNOYING / HORRIBLE / LOUSY. But you're [CIRCLE ALL] RESILIENT / INCREDIBLE / A TOTAL SMOKE-SHOW, and we know you can—and will!—get through this.

So take a deep breath, buy yourself a(n) [AMOUNT] of [TREAT], and remember that this isn't going to last forever.

You got this.

FOR WHEN _____

A DIY Tiny Pep Talk for When Something Exciting Is Happening

Hell yeah, [CIRCLE ONE] CHAMP / DIVA / SUPERSTAR / YOU !

We're so thrilled to hear about [EXCITING THING] ! There's no way around it: [EXCITING THING] is amazing, but it's also potentially [CIRCLE ONE] SCARY / STRESSFUL / NAUSEATING / GOING TO CHANGE EVERYTHING . Don't worry, even the most triumphant among us (like you, Tony Soprano, and Olympic figure skaters who just landed the triple axel) can use the occasional pep talk. So here goes.

You deserve all good things because you're [CIRCLE ALL] TALENTED / HARDWORKING / A TOTAL SMOKESHOW . Whatever emotions you're feeling about this [CIRCLE ONE] GOOD / GREAT / ABSOLUTELY INCREDIBLE achievement, you've earned this. We're proud of you.

So take a deep breath, buy yourself a(n) [AMOUNT] of [TREAT] , and remember that this moment isn't going to last forever, so enjoy it.

You got this.

PAULA SKAGGS and **JOSH LINDEN** are Chicago-based writers, comedians, cocreators of the game No Wrong Answers: Cards for Better Conversations, and cohosts of *Being Earnest (A Very Sincere Podcast)*.